Turn the Lights On;
I Can't Hear You

Ashlee Holland

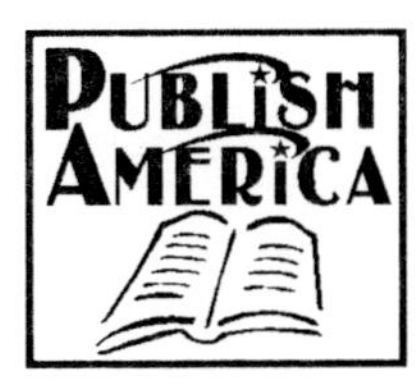

PublishAmerica

Baltimore

First printing

ISBN: 1-60441-953-9
PUBLISHED BY PUBLISHAMERICA, LLLP
www.publishamerica.com
Baltimore

Printed in the United States of America

Dedication

I would like to dedicate my book to the following women for educating, inspiring, and believing in me:

Sandy James Fox
Jane Driscoll
Joan Crawford
Trish Keller
My mother, Cindy Holland

Acknowledgments

I want to say thank you to Johnathan Barksdale and his family, to my best friends and my family for all the moral support through my deaf journey. My love to our daughter, Makayla Rose.

Introduction

Have you ever imagined what life is like without sounds? Listening to every second of our life whether we are crossing the crosswalk in New York City, hiking in the desert hearing a rattle snake, sleeping in our bed and hearing one of our children going to the bathroom and taking a shower, our boss's wearing brand-new shoes as she walks down in the hallway making noises while we are typing notes on the computer, and hearing ourselves and others breathing and eating food. It is all part of our hearing world. We can understand our loved ones' emotions as they go through phases in their lives, whether they are experiencing a broken heart or getting a promotion at work by hearing in their tone of voice how they feel about everything through their life time. Every day in this world requires hearing and sight to have an ability to know what is coming at us to avoid accidents and difficulties. If you cannot hear and are standing in the dark, you would understand about an urge to turn on the lights in order to "hear," as seeing what is going on, whether lip reading or watching others' doing actions that involved sounds, lets deaf people know what is going on.

There are many people out there who cannot imagine what we deaf people go through. There are even people out there that do not know people actually can have no hearing or some hearing. They are puzzled by this. In this silent world I have felt alone or shut off to go into my own world as I sit in the crowd watching people exchanging stories as they are too busy to include me. I have gotten used to these feelings, as I have been deaf since birth; I have been through a lot of obstacles that tested me for who I am today, my weakness, my strengths, and my identity that I shall accept. It took me awhile to figure out how to accept myself, so I no longer care about what people think of me or how they don't have the power to control me because my personal experiences have brought me up to the point where I have accepted and learned to love myself, and I deserve better.

I think people experience things for a personal reason, whether they fall in the pattern, like Alice in Wonderland falling down the rabbit hole, where saw all sorts of things happening; we say that we will not experience it, because we do not want to, yet it happens to us. So this could be a guide for you to grasp and understand what it is like to stand on our own feet with no sounds while continuing to live a life like others do where they rely on sounds. Also, just because we cannot hear, there are people who go through where they feel alone, whether struggling to live with an alcoholic at home, being abused, being overweight and teased by others, pressured to be skinny by others, having a learning disability, or being homeless. There is something that we all have in common: battling life, being heard and educated by the world's challenges for us to achieve while understanding what other people go through.

My goal for this book is to educate parents, teachers, families, or anyone in the community who is willing to learn about this silent world of ours while mentoring deaf children and adults to succeed and help them with the things that they go through, as they are not the only ones, because I also have been there; we wear the same pair of shoes.

"You must live in the present, launch yourself on every wave, find your eternity in each moment." —Henry David Thoreau

Famous Deaf People

Do you wonder if there are any deaf people out in the world who are well known for their remarkable talents or if they can do anything at all? Absolutely! There are several people who are successful at life and what they do who don't pit their deafness in first place to show people. They proved everyone wrong, showing that they have talents as well. Of course, being deaf is the main thing of who we are as a character. There are deaf people who also show off their deafness to be a role model for the silent world, where they have gone on several tours and been involved with foundations to help and be there for deaf children. There are people who have made their place in history that people would never have thought of, such as excelling at sports, beauty pageants, acting, singing, and several different kinds of roles out there. They have proved to all of us that they have made a wish on a star, and it came true where they have been motivated and driven to success, and not let the hearing world postpone their dreams at all. I have listed some famous deaf people. I know there are more people out there who are deaf and famous; I cannot put everyone here in this book or it will become a size of a library.

Art

Louis Frisino
He was born in 1934; he was deaf since birth. While growing up he enjoyed art and went to Maryland School for the Deaf. After graduating from high school he went to Maryland Institute of Arts. He specialized in realistic-looking animals such as ducks, dogs, and fish. His artwork was on stamps from Maryland back in 1987.

Granville Redmond

Granville was born in Pennsylvania on March 9, 1871. He had hearing until he lost it due to scarlet fever at the age of three. His family made a commitment by moving him and rest of the family from the East Coast to the West Coast for his education to be pursued at Berkeley School for the Deaf. After high school he went to California School of Design, where he worked along with several other artists. He got a scholarship to study in Paris at Academic Julian. Gottardo Piazzoni and Chaplin were among his lifelong friends. They studied American Sign Language to communicate with him. Chaplin had Granville teach him ASL and body language for his silent movies; Granville was cast in his seven silent films.

Douglas Tidlen

Douglas was born on May 1, 1860. He lost his hearing at the age of five due to scarlet fever, so he went to California School for the Deaf. He became a sculptor and moved to France for a while to pursue his talents in art. He was involved and was vice president of the World Federation of the Deaf and president of the California Association of the Deaf. People thought his work was similar to Michelangelo's or that he seemed talented like him, so they called him, "Michelangelo of the West."

Deaf and Blind

Julia Brace

Julia was born on June 3, 1807 in Newington, Connecticut. She had hearing and sight until she was five, when she was diagnosed with typhus fever. This left her deaf and blind. Soon she stopped speaking and learned home signs with her family as they communicated. She went to boarding school with kids who had hearing and sight, then she transferred to American School for the Deaf shortly before she turned eighteen. Back then, the school was named, Hartford Asylum for the Deaf and Dumb. She became famous for her skills and just being herself as a deaf and blind woman. She helped Dr. S.G. Howe to teach Laura Bridgeman. He learned by observing Julia at school and in her daily life.

Laura Bridgman

She was the first deaf and blind student of Dr. Samuel Howe at the Perkins School for the Blind.

Helen Keller

Helen Keller was born in 1880. At the age of nineteen months old she was diagnosed with scarlet fever or meningitis that left her deaf and blind. Her mother had sought help and asked Charles Dickens to help her to meet with Alexander Graham Bell, who was working with deaf children at the time. He set her up with Anne Sullivan, who became Helen's companion for 49 years. She taught her to communicate while dealing with her frustration as she was growing up. Helen and Anne traveled to 39 countries together. Also, Helen was the first deaf-blind person to graduate from college; she earned a bachelor's degree in 1904. Due to her talents, she was an advocate for people with disabilities, a suffragist, a pacifist, opposed Wilson, was a radical socialist and birth-control supporter. She managed to have time to write 12 books and published articles in magazines. She published books based on her personal experiences such as, *The Story of My Life, The World I Lived In, Out of Dark,* and *My Religion.*

Entertainment

Michelle Banks

She was born hearing but was diagnosed with spinal meningitis at an early age. She learned American Sign Language later on. She is a deaf actress, a founder and director of Only Theater, Inc. She played a role in the movie, *Malcolm X*. She also did a tour of *Reflections of a Black Deaf Woman*.

Linda Bove

She was born deaf to deaf parents and went to deaf schools through her educational life. She even went to Gallaudet College. She is an actress who she appeared as a librarian on *Sesames Street* from 1971-2003, where she introduced American Sign Language to kids. Also she appeared and played a role on Happy Days as a girlfriend of Fonzie.

Amy Ecklund

Amy was not born deaf. She lost her hearing at the age of six. She continued to speak, and later on she learned to read lips and use American Sign Language to communicate with others. She got a cochlear implant in 1999. For college, she earned a bachelor of fine arts degree. She was an actress for the TV soap opera, *Guiding Light*. She won several awards and was nominated for more.

Phyllis Frelich

Phyllis is considered to be one of the three deaf actresses in the 20th century who have done the most acting. She played a leading role in *Children of a Lesser God* on Broadway, where she won the 1980 Best Actress Tony Award. Marlee Matlin played her role in the film later on. She was born deaf, and her parents and rest of her eight siblings were all deaf. She was the oldest of her siblings. Not only did she play the role in *Children of a Lesser God*, she appeared in the TV shows, *E.R.* and *Diagnosis Murder*, and in the TV movie, *Love is Never Silent*, a Hallmark film. She continues to play small roles at the plays on Broadway.

C.J. Jones

C.J. Jones was born hearing to deaf parents. He lost hearing at the age of seven due to spinal meningitis. While growing up he was directing and playing roles in the plays before and after high school. Still to this day, he is still playing many hardworking roles in Hollywood and everywhere else in America. He is a CEO, producer, actor, director, comedian, and motivational speaker. He has had roles on *Frasier, Lincoln Heights, Sesame Street, Rainbow's End, Happy Hands Kids Klub, and Pathfinder.* His passion is the entertainment industry. He also wants to convey the message to deaf children and adults that "Being different does not mean being less worthwhile," according to his website, www.cjjoneslive.com.

Marlee Matlin

Marlee Matlin is considered as one of the most famous actresses today. She has played many roles and has been acknowledged for her hard work. She was born hearing to her parents, their third child. A year and half later she was diagnosed with roseola infantum. Even though she lost her hearing, she continued on with her life. She did plays at the age of seven to present. She played the major role in the movie, *Children of a Lesser God,* for which she won an Academy Award for Best Actress. Not only she had many acting roles, but she has found the time to travel to meet deaf children all over. She also is a spokesperson for National Captioning Institute. As spokesperson she advocated passing a law mandating that all TV have closed captioning. This law passed in 1995. This confident, amazing, talented woman once said of herself, "I have always resisted putting limitations on myself, both professionally and personally."

Anthony Natale

He is famous for appearing on the film, *Mr. Holland's Opus,* where his role was 15 minutes long. Also he appeared in *Jerry Mcguire,* where he was in the elevator signing with a girl, saying, "You complete me." He acted with Marlee Matlin in the suspense thriller, *Two Shades of Blue.* He made a documentary on how to learn sign language. During his free time he gives private lessons in sign language and how to be in shape. I do not know if he was born deaf if he became deaf. He has been deaf since his childhood, because he went to deaf schools before college.

Christy Smith

Christy Smith was born three months early and diagnosed with hearing loss since birth. Her mother helped her get speech therapy at a young age. While growing up she joined at Aspen Camp School for the Deaf and made deaf friends. She had a passion to go to the deaf high school in Washington, D.C., where later on she went to Gallaudet University and earned a degree. She appeared on *Survivor: Amazon* from October 2002-May 2003. After she got off *Survivor*, she had passion to help deaf children and inspired them by joining a television show that she produces, *Christy's Kids: Challenge Yourself,* for PBS.

Shoshannah Stern

She is well known for playing two roles that are non-hearing characters on shows. She was the first deaf person to play those roles. Shoshannah was born deaf, along with her siblings, who are deaf, as the 4th generation of deaf people in her family. She learned American Sign Language while she also learned how to lip read and speak while growing up. Also, she went to Gallaudet University to earn a degree. She has acted in *Weeds* and *Threat Matrix* for a few seasons.

Heather Whitestone

Many of you should know who Heather Whitestone is since she became the very first deaf Miss America in 1995. She lost her hearing eighteen months after her birth as a result of terrible reaction to diphtheria-tetanus vaccine. She was brought up in an oral world. Her family encouraged her to take dance classes at a young age, where one of her many talents showed. She absolutely loved dancing. She got into doing pageants in 1992, and went on to become Miss America.

She did not give up during those years. Actually, she did not know she won until the second runner up notified her. Since then she has developed an organization, STARS. She and her husband are both politically involved in other things. She did many tours around America. She strongly believed in oral language instead of sign language. Besides all the work she has done, she has published books, such as *Let God Surprise You: Trust God with Your Dreams.*

Ludwig van Beethoven

He is considered as one of the most talented musical composer in history. He studied Mozart and Hayden, and his father taught him music at a young age. After he turned 31 he lost some hearing, then at the age of 42 he became totally deaf. He continued playing his music pieces; research shows that he could still "hear" music because he could feel the vibration of the piano. He still composed music, but he did not perform in public very often after he lost his hearing.

Johnnie Ray

He was born in 1927. He had a mild hearing loss in his childhood; he wore one hearing aid at the age of fourteen. He is well known for his music. He produced songs such as, "Cry," and "The Little White Cloud that Cried." His very first film was the musical, *There's No Business Like Show Business.* He died in 1990.

Pete Townshend

Pete Townshend was born on May 19, 1945. He is famous for being a guitarist and songwriter for the band, The Who. During his time playing in the band and playing music on his time off, he lost his hearing because of the very loud volume of the music he performed and listened to on headphones. Because of his personal experience he helped to fund an organization called "Hearing Education and Awareness for Rockers."

Evelyn Glennie

Eveyln was born in 1965. She had hearing since birth, but began losing her hearing at the age of eight. By the time she reached the age of twelve she was profoundly deaf. While growing up, she played harmonica and clarinet. She attended the Royal College of Music; shortly after that she became the very first solo percussionist. She is a full-time solo percussionist, performing to large crowds all over the world. She feels people should look at her talents first instead of her deafness.

Leadership and Organizations

Kelby Brick

Kelby Brick is highly intelligent deaf man. He has an undergraduate degree from Gallaudet University and a law degree from Temple University. As an attorney he is an advocate for many legal issues concerning the deaf. Also he is involved in organizations such as National Association of the Deaf, and he was the director for The Law and Advocacy. Another achievement of his was co-writing the book, *Legal Rights: The Guide for Deaf and Hard of Hearing People.*

Juliette Gordon Low

Juliette began to lose her hearing at the age of seventeen and became progressively more deaf over the years of her adulthood. She was born in 1860 in Georgia. She was sent to a school in Virginia, where Thomas Jefferson's granddaughters taught her and other students. Later on in her schooling years she transferred to a school in New York. After falling in love and getting married to William Mackay Low, they moved to England, where she soon to discover her passion in the Girl Guide Association. She got so involved that it was a huge part of her life; she visited America some time later in her life and went to her hometown, Savannah. She opened her first Girls

Guide troop there. After six months it expanded to six troops. During 1913 she flew back to Savannah to check on the troops. They Girl Guides changed their name to Girl Scouts of America.

Rocky Stone
He lost his hearing during his teen years, and he became blind later on in his life. With blindness and deafness, he made a decision to get a cochlear implant to give it a try. In 1979, he was the Founder of Hearing Loss Association of America as "Self Help for Hard of Hearing People" where it is abbreviated as SHHH. Due to his personal experiences, he was very involved in Cochlear Implant Association, International Federation of Hard of Hearing People, and National Institute. Meanwhile, during his lifetime, he was with Central Intelligence Agency for 25 years. He wrote a book, *Living with Hearing Loss.* He passed away on August 13, 2004.

Dummy Hoy
He was born in 1862. He lost his hearing at the age of three due to meningitis. During his adult years he opened up a shoe-repair store and played baseball over the weekends on his time off from the store. His real name was Williams Ellsworth Hoy. During his time, people used the word "dumb" to mean "mute, unable to speak." It did not necessarily mean, "stupid," the primary meaning that we think of now. However, even then, some people used "dumb" to mean both unable to speak and stupid. Therefore, he was given the unkind nickname, "Dummy." He became famous for being the very first deaf professional baseball player in history. He passed away in 1961.

Curtis Pride
Curtis has been deaf since birth due to rubella; he grew up oral; he had lost 95% of his hearing and was excellent in lip reading. He became the second deaf professional baseball player in history along with Dummy Hoy. He and his wife have been actively involved with "Together with Pride," an organization to help kids with hearing aids.

Kenny Walker

Just like several famous people who have lost their hearing to illness when they were babies, he lost his hearing at the age two due to meningitis. He had a short career as a professional football player. He retired and became a football coach at the Iowa School for the Deaf.

Rush Limbaugh

Rush Limbaugh is well known for his work as an American radio talk-show host. He talks about politics. His fans love his work and his aggressive style. Later in his life he had a sudden loss of hearing due to a very rare autoimmune inner-ear disease. When dealing with this new challenge in his life, he learned how to continue to live his life daily with it. For work assistance, he uses Teleprompters and staff with phone calls at work while he hosts his radio program. He also got a cochlear implant to improve his hearing ability.

Types of Hearing Loss

Do you wonder if all deaf people just hear music and other things out in the world by just feeling sound vibrations, and is all hearing loss the same? Absolutely not. There are different levels for hearing loss, and everyone is different, responding to things at different times or ways. Think you will never lose your hearing because you were born hearing? Maybe someday you will lose your hearing due to damage in your environment whether loud working equipment you are using, being in a rock band, or you are just simply aging and losing your hearing slowly. My grandfather respected me more after he had a hearing loss just from aging. He did not wear hearing aids until he was in his mid 80s. By the time he wore hearing aids he would come up to me and give me his reports on what he could hear and could not hear, what bothered him, and how he could hear the warning beeps when the batteries were going to die.

Watching other people not responding to things on time or at all, you start to wonder if they have a hearing loss. But you don't want to say anything until you know the definite thing to prove that they have a hearing problem. There are several different ways to tell in children and adults by the way they handle things. The signs to look out for in children are:

They do not respond to you (not including when they don't respond on purpose),

Their speech is unlike other people's, in that they do not pronounce things clearly and at a normal speed—they talk slower than a normal rate,

They cannot hear the television or music; they might sit up in the front or close to it to hear it or complain about not being able to hear it,

They frequently say, "Huh?" when responding to conversations when they are confused because they did not hear the whole thing.

With adults, you can tell they might be becoming deaf when:

They don't get to the door after the doorbell rings,
They don't answer the telephone when it rings,
They turn up the volume on television or the radio so much that other people complain about how loud it is in the room,
They often ask people to repeat what they said until they understand,
They do not laugh at jokes or stories, as they miss the point of it because they could not hear the tone and what happened,
They ask others for notes at the lecture or an important event as they struggle to hear everything,
They get frustrated out in public when, because of distracting noises, they cannot hear what people say.

First, let's start out with basic education on hearing loss. There are three different types; they are *conductive hearing loss*, *sensorineaural hearing loss*, and *mixed hearing loss*. Remember that loss can occur because of a malformation or misfunction of a part of an individual's specific auditory system, for example there can be missing parts in the ear, or loss or lack can be genetic, inherited, present in a person's family tree.

Conductive hearing loss is where people have an ability to hear faint sounds; this is where they can be treated by surgeries or medications. What causes conductive hearing loss? The most common cases involve fluids in the middle ear from allergies or colds, ear infections, or benign tumors.

Sensorineural hearing loss is where people can hear faint sounds, but they have a difficult time understand speech and hearing things clearly. This cannot be treated with medication or surgery because there is damage to the inner ear, which is the cochlea, or to the nerves from the retro cochlear to the brain. The cause of this can be birth defects, birth injuries, diseases, genetic syndromes, tumors, head trauma, aging, and viruses. This is permanent hearing loss that cannot be fixed.

Mixed hearing loss is where people lose hearing in the inner and outer ear. It results from damage in the auditory nerve or cochlea.

Ever wonder what someone's hearing loss is or how much you can hear? People go to an audiologist to take an audiogram that informs them what exactly they have as hearing loss whether it is mild or severe loss. Then they get specific types of hearing aids that match the specific type of hearing loss if they want to wear hearing aids to hear sounds in their environment.

Normal range to no impairment	0 dB to 20 dB
Mild Loss	20 dB to 40 dB
Moderate Loss	40 dB to 60 dB
Severe Loss	60 dB to 80 dB
Profound Loss	80 dB or more

Mild Hearing Loss

With this type of loss, people have some difficulty keeping up with conversations, especially in noisy surroundings. Sometimes they do not wear a hearing aid for this loss.

Moderate Hearing Loss

With this type of loss, people have difficulty keeping up with their environment if there are distracting loud noises. Carrying on a conversation is difficult, especially if they do not use their hearing aids.

Severe Hearing Loss

With this type of loss people often wear hearing aids that match their specific loss; they may rely on lip reading and can use sign language as a communication. They definitely do not hear a lot of sounds without a hearing aid.

Profound Hearing Loss

People with this type of loss communicate with others through lip reading or sign language because they do not have enough hearing to hear without hearing aids. They do not hear exact sounds going on in the environment such as birds calling, whistling, water dripping, and other quiet sounds.

Normal range or no impairment obviously means that people can hear just perfectly fine in their environment. Mild loss is just slightly having a difficult time catching every word in conversations while Moderate loss is where they struggle a little bit more than mild hearing loss. Severe loss is having difficulty, and a person needs to lip read people during conversations, cannot hear at all without hearing devices on, and has a speech impairment. Profound loss has no hearing; people cannot hear at all even with devices.

"More than three million American children have hearing loss. An estimated 1.3 million of these children are under three years of age. Parents and grandparents are usually the first to discover hearing loss in a baby because they spend the most time with them. If at any time you suspect your baby has a hearing loss, discuss it with your doctor. He or she may recommend evaluation by an otolaryngologist—head and neck surgeon (ear, nose, and throat specialist)." This information came from www. Entnet.org website. If interested, you can check out the website for further readings.

If adults and children are losing their hearing as they are growing up, and they feel scared and frustrated because they cannot hear as much as they used to before, they can get help from all kinds of sources in their community. Help can include getting a hearing aid that helps them to regain their skills when using it; meeting people who go through similar things and can give out advice; making arrangements, whether at work, home, or school for them to continue with their daily lives; and with personal devices that make them feel secure. There are several ways to get help and feel comforted without freaking out and feeling miserable. I never had an opportunity to hear the normal range and will never be able to. I am doing great on my part, so if I can survive, so can you.

How to Communicate with Deaf People

There are several different ways to communicate with people who have different levels of hearing loss. It is important to learn how to communicate properly without offending people, without causing or feeling frustration, and without miscommunication. Whether it is one-on-one or group conversation, it is key to face the person with respect and even show enthusiasm to make them feel that they are included. Therefore, let's try to imagine what it feels like to be left out or to struggle to be part of a group. I hope these examples can help you at least imagine or bring memories of what you went through.

Example One: You are sitting in a large table at a restaurant with 12 people. You are sitting on the end of the table where at least four to six people are sitting in the middle. They are laughing and exchanging stories. They are pointing it out to you, asking you if you remember the events. To remember, you obviously have to understand at least half of what they said. You feel left out, as you have a person to talk to in front of you, and you wonder what other people are talking about.

Example Two: You are going to the movies where you cannot understand every word because of loud noises in the background of the movie. Would that frustrate you? Watching *American Idol* or a football game on TV, if you wish you can rewind over and over again to hear what they said to understand it, but you can't do that in a movie theater.

Example Three: You are going to a lecture where you are sitting in the very last rows of the auditorium. You struggle to hear everything in the person's speech because you are either too far away or the person has a voice that is too quiet to reach you.

Example Four: You are sitting in the car with your friends cruising around the town or on a road trip. You cannot hear at all except vibration of music. You can lip read your friends, but it is dark outside and inside of the car. You cannot see anyone's lips. You see your friends laughing and chatting away without you as you sit in your seat looking out in the window waiting for sunlight rays to come before you ask you friends to turn on the lights because you cannot hear them.

Example Five: You are outside doing gardening work, such as mowing the grass and using the leaf blower to blow all the leaves away. Your partner comes up to you and starts talking to you. You hear their voice as muffled sounds. You have to turn your equipment off and start the conversation all over again.

Now, let's stop imagining all these examples and move forward on how to communicate with deaf people. First, face the person in front of you and speak clearly at a moderate speed. Do not speak so slowly that you could be singing the ABC's song in a slow motion; it will rather be distracting and offensive. Do not talk with food in your mouth, as they will focus on the annoying way you chew your food; besides your family taught you manners during your childhood! Also, do not put your hand to hold your chin up or use hand gestures around your face while you are talking because we cannot read lips while you are using your hands over your face as if you are covering your pimples!

Depending on the hearing loss and how they communicate, there are people who can lip read but use American Sign Language to communicate back. The definition of sign language from the dictionary: "Also called sign. Any of several gestural systems of communications, esp. employing manual gestures, as used among deaf people." And again another part of definition is: "Any means of communication, as between speakers of different languages, using gestures."

A majority of the deaf community use American Sign Language; it is a visual, quiet, and accepting language, where everyone can feel that they have the art of the communication without getting lost or feel left out. It is not difficult to learn the language. My deaf friend Kate taught many rafting guides at a rafting company where we worked over the summer in California. They learned very quickly and seemed to enjoy it thoroughly. I grew up oral. She introduced me to another side of the deaf's world, which is American Sign Language, so I went back home to Arizona as the season ended and took sign language Classes with my best friend, Brooke. I thought it was far beyond amazing, and fun, because I finally felt I was part of everything. I can give you an example; we were out on the river going rafting, and we could not hear, because you have to take your hearing aids out, as they are not waterproof. As we were rafting and going down the rapids, the guides would sign to us as we were, like, 20 feet away, giving us warnings about the rapids, how to paddle properly, or carrying on conversations. Here we are understanding the language without relying on a voice across a noisy river. It helped me a lot while it made me feel secure.

Just remember, this language requires facial expressions, just as in all kinds of verbal or visual communication you use with others. Facial expressions are a huge part of communication because it sends vibes on how the person is feeling. I have met people who smiled all the time, as if they were proud of their beautiful, white, straight teeth. They smiled so much all the time that I could not figure out if they were sharing good or bad stories, like smiling and saying, "My Grandfather died last night!" If I did not understand their words completely, I would think the person was happy because of no appropriate facial expressions, and I would nod. But if the person acted very sad and said, "My grandfather died last night," I would feel the sadness through seeing their facial expressions. Their facial expressions would give me helpful clues about what they were saying. I would want to understand what they said, because I would want them to know I was there for them.

If you are interested in learning about American Sign Language to use it to communicate with a friend, employer, boss, family member, or partner you can take lessons from websites, borrow books from the library, and go to a local community for class such at colleges or churches. If you know someone who is deaf and is fluent in sign language, you can have that person set up a class to teach you and your friends who are interested in learning with you, as it could be a positive, fun learning experience!

Another type of communication with other people is pen and paper as they jot things down. For an example, they take a pen and paper or small whiteboard with a marker with them to a restaurant or dentist appointment. They write things down like what they want to eat for lunch or questions they want to ask the dentist. Normally, they understand what other people are saying, and if not at the point, they write it down to answer their question.

We express our thoughts to others and understand each other and our needs by communication. We want ourselves and other individuals to be heard through our voices as we make a statement. We are connected by communication. Reading each others' minds through our body language, is a thread of communication. Learning to meet to each other's needs and understanding each other's backgrounds, where we come from, is done by learning to communicate with others. Success and confidence are created by communication as we learn how to approach others in life by using these tools. There are famous writers and speakers who talked about communication. I have included some here:

"When we have the courage to speak out—to break our silence—we inspire the rest of the 'moderates' in our communities to speak up and voice their views." ~Sharon Shuster

"Be sincere; be brief; be seated." ~Franklin Delano Roosevelt

"When people talk, listen completely. Most people never listen." ~Ernest Hemingway

"Nothing is so simple that it cannot be misunderstood." ~Freeman Teague, Jr.

"Our prime purpose in this life is to help others. And if you can't help them, at least don't hurt them." ~Dalai Lama

"If the person you are talking to doesn't appear to be listening, be patient. It may simply be that he has a small piece of fluff in his ear." ~Winnie the Pooh

"And the deaf soul struggles, strains forward, to lip-read what it needs: And something is said, quickly, in words of cloud-shadows moving and the unmoving turn of the road, something not quite caught…" ~Denise Levertov

"I've learned that people will forget what you said, people will forget what you did, but people will never forget how you made them feel." ~Maya Angelou

"Words mean more than what is set down on paper. It takes the human voice to infuse them with shades of deeper meaning." ~Maya Angelou

How Do Deaf People Hear?

What devices do deaf people use to hear? There are few common devices. It depends on their hearing loss and what they opt for. The most common devices are hearing aids, and processors for cochlear implants.

How do people get a hearing aid? Normally, they go to an audiologist to have a test, an audiogram. Then the audiologist helps them decide what kind of a hearing aid is a best match to their hearing loss level. Here are several different types of hearing aids for all ranges of hearing loss.

What is a cochlear implant? A cochlear implant is a surgically implanted device that restores hearing for some people with severe to profound hearing loss. Cochlear implants help patients to build abilities in their daily lives. For example, they help people improve their career skills, education skills, social skills, and many other kinds of skills that they use every day. The difficult challenges that they face as deaf people every day are not that difficult anymore because they have a technology that can help them to hear, and therefore, communicate more effectively with more people, and understand more of what is going on around them. Cochlear Implants provide the best technology for deaf people to be part of the hearing world. Many deaf people opt not to have a cochlear implant for personal reasons. One of the main reasons is that they are in the deaf culture and feel fine with themselves.

Cochlear implants are not a miracle technology that changes everything overnight. They work over a period of time, because it takes a while to improve the hearing loss. A cochlear implant does not reverse the damage that causes some loss of hearing. It does not work when the device is off; it only works when the device is turned on and activated. After patients get a cochlear implant and get their device turned on, it is unpredictable because the results are different for each cochlear-implant patient. Cochlear implants use an electric wire to help stimulate hair cells to move faster to receive enough information. When people are deaf, their hair cells in their ears are damaged, resulting in defective sound. So audiologists program each cochlear implant device. They monitor the programs in the devices to assure their effectiveness and make the sound comfortable.

There are criteria that the deaf must meet to be approved to be cochlear implant candidates. They must have a severe-to-profound hearing loss. Because they have to have a severe-to-profound hearing loss, it helps them to improve their skills. If a hearing person has lost some hearing, they are not good candidates to have a cochlear implant because they will hear too much. Their routines and hobbies will be destroyed and they will be distracted because they hear too much. Candidates must be motivated and committed to the use of the cochlear implant in order to receive maximum benefits. Also, candidates must have a good family and friends to have their support to help them to motivate to improve their hearing loss. The FDA, audiologists, and surgeons do not want to implant a patient where their skills are inappropriate. A patient who is not motivated enough, is lazy, or is disorganized will not benefit, and it would be a waste for them to get an implant. Toddlers and adults are the best age groups to gain approval for obtaining a cochlear implant. Also, one of the requirements is that patients undergo some medical screening, such as having CT scans, medical exams, and audiograms to qualify. Doctors won't perform the surgery until they do CT scans and others because they have to determine the condition of the patients' bones and find out about other health problems.   Patients must have realistic expectations for the cochlear implant. Audiologists and medical care givers ensure that they do have obtainable expectations. When they have expectations that are too high, they will head toward negativity and will be disappointed quickly. So candidates must review the risk, consequences, and the amount of training they will need in order to decrease the high expectations. It is not easy to get approval for a cochlear implant from FDA Regulations, audiologists, and surgeons, and it takes awhile to get approval.

Cochlear implants have a device that patients must wear. They wear an external device called a processor that is located on the outside of the skull behind the ear. It has a microphone, computer, and connecting cables. The microphone helps to receive the sounds, including speech that is occurring in that environment. Computer and connecting cables help to get the programs going and improves on speech. When patients go in their audiologist's office to get their device programmed, they are usually surprised at what they first hear. It usually doesn't match what they thought speech would sound like. They think speech sounds like a robot. But after listening to the processor for a while, they usually do not think it sounds like a robot anymore. They gradually hear like a normal hearing person hears after going through training and programming.

Hearing-impaired people normally wear a hearing aid to help them to hear the sounds and speech around them. Hearing aids and cochlear implants are completely different from each other. Hearing aids have different sound quality than the cochlear implant. Hearing aids are not electric, while cochlear implants are electric. Although they both help hearing-impaired people hear, their sound qualities are different. Hearing aids receive loud sounds, such as pounding on the doors, hammering on walls, dishes dropping on floors, doors slamming, and airplanes flying by. Also, loud speech in another term is called high frequency. High frequency receives "m," "b" and "d." Soft sounds are water running, birds singing, papers rustling, music playing, and dogs walking. Soft speech, which is low frequency, includes "s," "ch," "t," "sh," and many vowels. Hearing aids are one piece of equipment. Cochlear implants have one piece of equipment located on the inside of the skull, and the other piece is located on the outside of the skull. Meanwhile, cochlear implants have better sound quality then hearing aids. Hearing aids do not receive enough information to help profound hearing loss, although, the technology of hearing aids is drastically improving all the time to help deaf people with a profound-to-severe hearing loss. At last, the results with these two different technologies for hearing-impaired people to use are different. The researches show that patients hear different sounds, and they respond at different times with different sounds.

There are risks in getting cochlear implants that candidates might experience. The risks are surgery risks. Patients' surgery usually takes at least three to eight hours. Then they can go home on the same day of the surgery. Doctors prefer to implant in the ear where it has a better hearing the other side, so the cochlear implant works better and faster. Surgery risks include dizziness, neck pains, headaches, numbness, and itchiness. After the surgery, the surgery site takes at least six weeks to heal.

There are opponents of cochlear implants and there are arguments over cochlear implants. One of the arguments is that the hearing environment and deaf culture are against parents' decisions on and implanting these in their children. Since the best times to implant the devices are when a child is very young or when a person is an adult, parents make the choice for their children. The children do not get to choose. The laws say that it is the parents' right to decide. Parents often have a hard time deciding about cochlear implants. One of their tough decisions is based on whether they should include their child partially into the hearing world. Parents also must make sure that they and their deaf child are committed to the training and wearing the device. They have to make sure they are willing to experience the future harassment from the deaf culture and opponents if they decided to get a cochlear implant for their child. (Sometimes people against implants can give people with cochlear implants a hard time about having one.) In some cases, adults who were implanted as kids choose not to wear the device anymore. They decide to go silent. Deciding on going silent is hard for young candidates because they hear too much and did not have a choice whether they wanted it or not when they were young. It is one of the biggest problems with parents and cochlear implant candidates.

Many people, particularly in the deaf culture, feel that people shouldn't get implants until they are old enough to make a decision themselves. Deaf adults get to choose if they want a cochlear implant. Young children should not decide because they are too young to understand the risks and commitment of the cochlear implant. FDA regulations, audiologists, and surgeons get to decide on final implant after the parents review information. This argument is called autonomy. Autonomy means self-governing or self-directing choices. If parents make the choice for their children, their children cannot act autonomously; they cannot choose for themselves. Opponents of cochlear implant believe that parents are controlling, and the children are helpless because they do not get to choose. Also, the opponents believe parents rush into decisions with a lack of information. Accordingly, there are two different communities for hearing-impaired people. The deaf culture is where deaf people do not speak orally or wear cochlear implants. They use sign language as their language.

The hearing-impaired culture consists of hearing-impaired people who speak orally and wear hearing devices or cochlear implants to be part of the hearing world.

The deaf culture is against cochlear implants. They believe cochlear implants ruin the deaf culture, taking people away from it to be part of the hearing world. They fear that their culture will fail because of the cochlear implant that deaf people choose to use. Consequently, they feel threatened because of the increase use of cochlear implants. ASL is a sign language (it stands for American Sign Language) that is used by the deaf people and is the primary language of deaf culture. For them ASL is easier and not stressful for the deaf culture because it is very visual. Because most people in the hearing culture do not know ASL, and the deaf culture tends not to use communication that would bring them into the hearing culture, they remain unique with a culture of their own. They do not want to be part of the hearing world. Gallaudet College is a college for the deaf people; they educate students who speak in ASL. The deaf community argues that children who are young and deaf should choose whether they want to communicate by using ASL or to communicate in English. This choice largely determines which culture a person who is deaf will live in.

The rehabilitation process is one of the main issues in cochlear implants. It is a huge amount of commitment that a cochlear implant candidate will have to make. Cochlear implant patients put much energy into training skills. The training includes speech and listening skills. Also, auditory training with cochlear implant candidates is more successful than with non-cochlear-implant candidates. The results are that the cochlear implant candidate does a better job with speech and listening skills. They accomplish more because they want to hear better and have better technology to aid them as they undergo training. They improve in listening skills and speech skills with the environment that is surrounding them. Non-cochlear-implant candidates do not go through the same amount of training as the cochlear implant candidates do. Cochlear implant patients undergo programming and training with the device. Patients will benefit from regular auditory training sessions. It is not easy for medical care givers and audiologists to predict the improvement each patient with a cochlear implant will have because it is based on how much effort and commitment the cochlear implant candidate puts in. Each cochlear implant candidate hears differently. Some must lip-read with their cochlear implant while other do not have to lip-read. Each one of the candidates' accomplishments and goals are based on motivation and commitments. It takes time to hear better through training. The training and listening help to teach the brain the sounds of speech all over again so that it hears and comprehends it.

Therefore, some individuals choose to get a cochlear implant to improve their hearing loss. Hearing-impaired individualities that choose to get a cochlear implant to improve their hearing loss want to be part of the hearing world. Cochlear implants have been successfully used for over 20 years. They the implants have improved, and the rate of those getting them has been growing. The improvements with the cochlear implant patients are that 80% of patients are mainstreamed in classrooms in grades K-12. Another improvement with the cochlear implants is that 80% of children and adults are able to talk on the phone. The cochlear-implant patients who can listen on the phone still struggle. The researches show that cochlear implant patients do a better job than they did with a hearing aid before they go implanted. For example, their audiogram has been improved with listening and speech tests that they participated in. Also, they improved the abilities that they used daily; they are able to hear more than ever before. The companies, audiologists, and hearing world believe that children who are implanted have improved speech and grammar skills. Normally, hearing-impaired children have poor speech and grammar skills because they cannot hear that their brain does not pick up fast enough. Cochlear implant candidates feel more confidence about themselves and their daily routines when using their implant. They are more aware of what is going on around them, and that helps them feel secure.

To this end, cochlear implants provide the best technology for deaf people to be part of the hearing world and improve their abilities. Their challenges are not that difficult anymore after being implanted.

My Side of Silent World with Cochlear Implant and Hearing Aids

When I was a year and half old I had to wear hearing aids. I had to wear two pouches to carry them in. It looked like I was wearing a walkman player with ear phones. I absolutely hated it, except for all the cute pouches that my mother bought for me to match my outfits. Then few years later, I received an updated hearing aid, the behind-the-ear kind. I like it a lot better than my very first hearing aids. However, one day, my family and I went to Great Escape Amusement Park in Lake George, New York for the day. It was an hour-and-a-half drive. On the night before we went to Great Escape I always got as excited as if Santa Clause was coming. My mother realized that I did not have my hearing aids on after a few rides on the roller coaster, so my family assumed that it fell out during the aggressive rides. They decided to go through all the garbage cans, and could not find them. That night we went home, and my brother found my hearing aids under the pillow seats of the couch where we were playing "Forts," as I hid them under there before we went to Great Escape. Oops!

There are several different types of hearing aids which are worn behind the ear or in the ear, and there are waterproof hearing aids. They all are at different price ranges. In-the-ear hearing aids used to be for people with mild hearing loss; today they are available for profound hearing loss. I recently went to see an audiologist and was amazed at how the technology has changed drastically in a short period of time! They are now so tiny that you cannot even tell when people wear them. I do not know why they do that for sure; I wonder if it is for comfort or to make people not feel self conscious about wearing bigger, more noticeable hearing aids.

While growing up, I had behind-the-ear kinds with ear molds. As I grew up, I had to get new ear molds very often, or else I would sound like a mouse squeaking by a cat when I smiled. Actually, one day in high school (this is very embarrassing for me to share) we all were sitting in my English Class during spring time. I remember we had the windows open, as it was very cool day, and we were talking about the play, *Romeo and Juliet*, as it was part of our assignment. We shared jokes in class, and I laughed often during them. Meanwhile, a girl sitting by me was freaking out as she thought there was a bee buzzing by her that came in from the window. Every time I was smiling, there she goes freaking out. Then I realized the sound was my hearing aid buzzing because I needed a new ear mold! I had to turn it off because I could not stop smiling and laughing during the lecture that our teacher gave us. He had to close the window, as everyone thought there was a bee in the classroom.

I met few deaf people while growing up. Some refused wear a hearing aid, and others refused to use American Sign Language, as they spoke orally. They felt ashamed to wear a hearing aid because they would be recognized by others as having a hearing loss. I always felt embarrassed to wear my hair up when I was in my teens because of crucial classmates who were judgmental and trying to be popular. But then I realized that it helped me hear and respond to things faster instead of just standing there while people were waiting for my attention as the clock ticked and tocked. I learned that it is about you and your needs, not about what other people think of you.

When I was growing up in Massachusetts, we would get a monthly newsletter about deaf people, hearing aids, and cochlear implants. As my mother read more about the cochlear implant, she asked me if I wanted it. I clearly remember to this day that I was lying on her bed when I was eight years old, wondering why she would ask me if I wanted a cochlear implant, as if I thought I was not good enough. I was eight and felt very normal. I did not want it at all. They stopped asking me about the cochlear then. After graduating from middle school my social life changed. When I was out playing with friends at nighttime, I struggled to lip read in the dark. I would have to ask friends to speak to me in the areas where there were the lights so I could see to lip-read. Not only that, I felt left out when swimming in the pool or when everyone else was talking on the phone and I could not perform the kinds of activities that hearing teenagers could do that required listening. I stood very silent; I felt very self conscious. I was nervous. How would my friends respond to me when I could not hear them swimming in the pool when we played games such as Marco Polo? With my very close friends, we had a system. When it was my turn, I would say, "Marco," with my eyes closed and wait for them to splash at me as a code instead of replying, "Polo." I absolutely despised the game, "Telephone." I had to sit out of that game whenever friends played it.

After all these teenager experiences, I decided to get a cochlear implant. So I met with an audiologist and surgeon when I was 14 years old. They had me to read books, go through several testing with MRI, CT scans and audiograms to see if I was qualified to have a cochlear implant. I had a lot of homework to do with them for at least six to eight months to be qualified. I was actually at the borderline with these decisions, as they were deciding if I should have a cochlear implant.

Finally, one early dawn in December 1999 before the Y2K crisis was going to not occur, I had a surgery. I cried the night before, when my brother, who was a senior in high school, came home to get stuff to go out with his friends. He comforted me, as I feared my whole life would be changed and not work out the way I wanted it to. My parents were extremely nervous with the procedures, as my childhood best friend, Ally, had a cochlear implant surgery in Boston that lasted almost six hours. I could not fall asleep with the meds they gave me until they wheeled me into the surgery room; I saw the surgeon preparing his tools for the surgery in front of me in this green-tiled room. Immediately I passed out for sure.

I woke up. My surgery had taken no longer than two and half hours. I saw all my family around me waiting for me to wake up for two hours. I remembered seeing my grandmother and mother sitting close to me and holding my hands. They rushed out to get rest of the family to come and see me. Meanwhile, I had bitten my tongue during the surgery, so that I had a swollen bump in my tongue while looking like Princess Leah from Star Wars as they had bandaged my ear. Being in horrific pain, as I could not sleep on my sides or turn while I was sleeping, I had pillows around my head. My mother had to help me to go to bathroom or shower. She had to help balance me while I was walking and standing.

I cried often and thought to myself, "What have I done?" It took at least two weeks for me to start going back to normal life. I had to go back to school, as my winter break was over. I was absolutely horrified with my hair, as they had shaved on the side of my ear with the hair around it; I still had hair on the top of my head that covered the missing area. My father took me to school on my first day back. I was extremely excited to go back and see friends. The next thing we knew, as we were pulling into the parking lot, a woman was driving 65 miles per hour and did not see us, so she hit us in the back of our van. I almost flew out of the window in front of me while my father hit his head on the dashboard. All the windows shattered, and the cold air rushed in. I was really scared and was in pain due to whiplash and was nervous about my recent surgery. Luckily, my teacher of the deaf saw us and called my mother at work to come down, as she was working within few blocks away from my school area. I saw her running toward us in her scrub uniform, all worried. The ambulance took me to the hospital. Can you believe I was at the hospital twice in two weeks? At least I got a cute teddy bear from cute gentlemen in the ambulance.

When you have a cochlear implant, you should always bring this identification card with you, as you cannot have MRI scans. If you are unconscious and they put you in the machine to scan you, you are most likely to suffer real damage or even worse, die, because of the magnet in your head. It will crush your skull due to the magnetic stuff inside of the machine. Be careful! It took me over a month to use my processor for the first time because they wanted me to recover completely. They wanted to take the staples out after they feel confident that I was ready to hear for the first time in the cochlear-implant world. Wow, don't I sound like a robot?

When I got home with the processor, I cried hysterically, because I was up in front of the television, and with the volume blasting all the way I still could not hear anything. When my mother clapped her hands, I absolutely would cringe at the sound of it. I had to go to therapy for at least few months to learn the sounds with my processor. I secretly did not wear it at high school while I was supposed to, just like I was supposed to wear glasses in school, and my teacher of the deaf would catch me and make me wear it. After several months of listening therapy and giving it a try I started to learn to enjoy it better than I had the very first night. A year later, I started to wear it all the time. I felt like I could not live without it. I still cannot live without it to this day.

When people asked me if I would recommend a cochlear implant to all the deaf people, I tell them it is up to them. It all depends on the culture and what they do with their lives, whether they are oral or use American Sign Language as communication. Other factors that matter are if they feel really left out and have low self esteem. I would warn them that it is very exhausting at first, and another thing is that it is a painful surgery to have. I would remind them that they have to be serious about it, as they cannot go back to wearing a hearing aid in the implanted ear, because the hair cells are destroyed. So they would have to wear the processor to hear things in life. It also takes time to adjust to the sound qualities. Everyone is different.

The down side of it is that they cannot go to Walgreen's to buy hearing-aid batteries for the processor; they have to order batteries on online or by phone order, because the batteries are made specially for the processor and program you use. My first processor contained two batteries a day every day; then I changed processors for an updated program with features that suited my deafness. After switching processors I went through three batteries every week, which was a huge difference while it had better sound quality in it. For the last eight years that I have been using the processor, I have loved it, but I do not enjoy dealing with new programs that the audiologist downloads every once in a while to update the sound quality to keep improving my hearing skills. I remember that I did like the programs few times, and other times I thought I did until I got outside of the building to walk to my car to go home. I heard different things out there from what I had heard in the quiet office with my audiologist. Sometimes I would get sad and panic because I had school or work to attend, where I was not completely confident with the new programs due to the sounds being different. I would write notes for a week where I felt there were things that sounded loud or too soft. I remembered one afternoon I drove to my boyfriend's house and sobbed all afternoon because I could not hear my favorite songs very well. He went with me to my appointments to make some adjustments with the sounds. Recently, they are coming up with a lot of ideas for processors like colors. They have improved their water resistance. They are not trying yet to make them 100% waterproof; they are just trying to protect them from a few splashes from the pool or rain. There are new devices to use it with telephone, television, and music. I can still have a difficult time with the cochlear implant because sounds fluctuate, and they are constantly changing and updating programs to help me improve my hearing skills. Sometimes I receive headaches from listening to many sounds, but I enjoy being able to hear the sounds that I could not imagine before.

For people who are looking into cochlear implants, there are few things that I would recommend. People should do their homework by reading books about it. They should meet local deaf people with cochlear implants in their town. (Their audiologists can help out with that.) They should share their questions and concerns with their audiologists and surgeons. They should think about their lifestyle, where they are with things in life. Do they have support from family and friends who will stand by them while they are going through therapy and healing time to learn to hear all over again?

I definitely would not be where I am at today if I did not have the support from my family and friends through the times I went through as I felt alone or struggling to learn to hear the sounds of birds, water running, crickets chirping, and other sounds. There are definitely sounds that bother me, even having listened to them for eight years now.

Here is advice for deaf people looking into hearing aids. I am definitely poor and cannot afford them. This sounds quite silly, but I had a hearing aid for two weeks after not having a hearing aid for a year. My puppy chewed it up; I could not face my parents after all they had done to help get a new hearing aid for me. So for almost two years I went without a hearing aid. I went to see a counselor at vocational rehabilitation and found out that they could help me with hearing aids, but he could not guarantee it, as they are expensive. He recommended that I call my health insurance to see if they provided hearing-aid coverage. They did, but I was too late. There were certain age requirements, and I was already over 21. I wished I knew that when I first got them, but I did not get this kind of opportunity to help my parents with hearing-aid finances. My deaf friend Kate received a hearing aid through Starkey's Hearing Foundation. She only had to pay $200.00 instead of several thousand dollars for it. So if they are in financial situations, people can always check out the local scholarships, ask their audiologists, go to vocational rehabilitation for assistance, and see if their health insurance covers it or anything else. You will be surprise how much you can find in your community and in your state!

Devices for Personal Use

Ever wonder how deaf people communicate in the hearing and deaf worlds? There are several ways to communicate with other human beings here on this world as the technology rapidly grows and changes. Over the years, the technology and devices keep improving drastically and offer even better opportunities for deaf people every day for them to use daily. The people who invent the technology think of ways for them to communicate for work, social life, and personal life at home. For work they can use these personal devices as they step out to the door to work and go to their office to make calls to contact people professionally. When they have friends and family members to hang out with, they go to events and use their cell phones to text, e-mail, relay, and use the Internet to arrange things. Living at home with their family or alone, if they are in college, they have home-assistance devices, where they do not have to rely on others for waking them up. If they are parents, devices can alert them to go check on their newborn baby. Devices can warn them to leave the house or call someone because the smoke detector just went off. There are things to alert people that the doorbell has rung.

Overall, they have many devices to use to be independent and not have to rely on others. As you read below, you will learn more about what kind of devices they use to be independent; you will become familiar with them, as you could receive phone calls at the office from these kinds of services from a deaf person. Meanwhile, just to remind you, please be careful how you portray yourself over the phone, as it is monitored. Deaf people can feel you are discriminating against them if you do not put up with their calls or if you show signs of disrespect.

Doing this can get your company in trouble.

Voice Carry Over Phone:
This type of phone offers an excellent opportunity for people who wants to use their voice on the phone but can struggle to hear loud noises. As they talk on the phone, they can always read the screen in front of them that relays messages if it is loud in their room or they did not get every word in the conversation. Also, they can print messages from their answering machine, so they do not have to rely on other hearing people to translate messages for them. There is another type of a phone that is very similar to Voice Carry Over Phone, which is called Cap Tel. It stands for Captioned Telephone.

IP Relay Services:
This is where a caller uses the Internet to call a hearing person. The operator translates conversations back and forth. First thing they do is explain what the relay services are and how to communicate by saying, "Go Ahead," when they are done talking at the moment. This is good for people who do not have TTY or Voice Carry Over Phone. It is fast and easy.

Video Relay Services:
This is for people use American Sign Language through the video instead of text services. They can see the person they are calling over the Internet with a video-equipment hook up. Also, when they receive messages they look at the screen where there is a local Telecommunication Relay Services operator where they, called a communication assistant. Deaf people can use this to call hearing people as well. They like to use this because they can see the facial expressions and body language through the screen instead of reading text, where they try to picture how the speaker is feeling at the moment.

TTY:

This stands for Text Telephone, and another name is TDD, which stands for Telecommunication Device for the Deaf. This type of phone does not require listening and speaking skills to communicate; it is all in text. It requires the opposite caller to use TTY as well. It prints the conversation as it goes. There is a screen on the machine on which you read the text. However, if a person is calling a person who does not have a TTY and still wants to use their TTY, they can use Telecommunications Relay Service, where an operator will translate with a TTY user and hearing person.

Relay Conference Captioning:

A person with hearing loss can use this kind of phone for meetings, conference calls, video conferences, and phone calls. Sprint and Federal Relay Services provide this type of technology. However, a person has to call and arrange within 48 hours for Captioner to be available to type captions on the screen while using and reading the Relay Conference Captioning technology. To help the captioner not to struggle with typing errors or get confused with names, events, and agenda, prior to meetings they can share information with the captioner.

Cell Phones:

There are different kind of cell phones out there that provide text messaging, AIM, which is Instant Messaging, Internet and e-mail. Blackberry, Sidekick, and other kinds of phones provide all of these services. Personally, I think a person with a hearing loss who wants to pursue this cell phone should sign up for a phone package that is unlimited. I had few cell phones and was signed up with unlimited or up to 200 texts per month. My bills were between 100 to 200 dollars a month. I have owned a sidekick for three years, and I have an unlimited package with all these types of communication for me to use. It is good for people who lead a busy life, with a job, traveling, relationships, and other personal things.

Doorbell Notification:
Doorbell Notification offers security in a house by alerting people with hearing loss when someone is at the door who rings the doorbell. It notifies them by flashes of light. Also, for people who do not have a doorbell they have Door Knocker. They have devices that are wireless sensors and Flashing Strobe Pager/Signalers that detect movement within 100 feet and alert by flashing the light.

Baby Cry Monitors:
Baby Cry Monitors signal deaf people when their child is crying by light flashing or vibration. Most of them come in wireless, so they can carry them around the house wherever they go.

Smoke Detector Alarm:
This device helps to alarm people when the smoke detectors go off. One version has a big light that flashes on the wall. Another version has a vibrator to wake people if they are sleeping.

Alarm Clocks:
There are several alarm clocks that help deaf people to wake up in the mornings by flashing a light or vibrating the bed. The vibrating alarm does not feel like the whole bed is shaking. If a person placed it under their pillow, a person would feel it. I have used it before, and my friends did not feel it when they were sleeping next to me.

There are several other devices for us to use and feel a part of the hearing world. We have the right to use these devices so we can be equal as others. I know different locales offer assistance for deaf people to use in particular situations to feel we are just like other hearing people in a way. If seeking into help with finances or assistance, check out what your state offers. Most of them provide assistance for people with needs as long as they set up an appointment and fill out an application. There are rules very particular rules for those who have been provided devices to follow. If you benefit from government assistance for one of these, be very careful to follow the guidelines.

Dogs Are Our Best Friends!

Literally, dogs are our best friends. Dogs are our joy and happiness, as they can comfort us through good and bad times by just simply cuddling with us. They definitely protect us from many things in our environment. Meanwhile, they can notify us that someone is on our property or in our surroundings outside, as they bark constantly until we check it out. They cheer us up and greet us when we return home at the end of our day. It is the best welcome we could have in our homes.

I have wanted a dog for years and years. My best friend, Ally, she had a couple of dogs while we were growing up in Beverly, Massachusetts. I often spent the nights at her house on weekends. Her dogs would play with us. I would go home and beg my mother to let us have a dog. I used to create a journal while I was growing up writing about cocker spaniels to convince my mother to buy me one. She claimed it would not work because would be too much work, and allergies run in the family.

So we moved to Arizona, and few years later, my brother and mother came home one evening while I was watching television with my father. They brought in this American Eskimo dog named Skeeter. My mom's patient had asked her if we wanted a dog. The dog was almost one year old. I seriously thought my brother was dog sitting Skeeter for a while until they informed me it was my dog. I considered it as a family dog to share the love with everyone! She is amazing; she is the first dog we have ever owned. I was fourteen years old when I got her; I noticed the difference, as she made me feel comfortable in my own home on my own when everyone was out at working. She would go up to the front door and bark. She was always right whenever someone was on our property lurking around, when cops were pulling people over, or someone was visiting us.

Then my brother got a dog from his girlfriend at the time. He could not have the dog at the apartment so he had his dog, Deisel, at my parents' house. To this day, Diesel is living with them. He protected me often from people and barked whenever someone was on our property. Then my best friends and I saved a dog off the highway. We looked for the owner for few weeks. The dog got used to me. She would cry whenever I left the room. She is very loyal to me, as she sleeps in bed with me until I get up. She would wait forever with no whining. She did not like many guys that came in our home. She would go under the table or walk away. If she enjoys someone she will show them affection. She always walks by me when we go for walks; she doesn't run off when I take her off the leash. She is really good to me and lets me know if something odd is going on in my environment. Then John and I got a puppy together. She is very active and playful. With no training she wakes us up when the alarm clock goes off, perhaps, since she wants us to wake up and play with her. If any other alarms go off in the house, she would go to them and wake our company up.

My friend Kate has had a yellow lab dog since he was a year old. I met her in Kernville, California. Cody, her dog, would sleep with her in the truck or in the tent whenever they are camping out. He was really her guard, as he was very protective of her. She would sign to him, "best friends," and he would give her his paw. When she would sign, "Sit," he immediately obeyed and sat. She signed to him with no voice. He is a very intelligent and well-behaved dog. I told her that he is my handsome prince!

There is a main website that offers information and assistance on dogs for the deaf people. It is http//dogsforthedeaf.org/. It is a terrific website; it says that they get dogs who are rescued from owners who don't want them. They train them to assist deaf people. If you check out your community, they should have programs and websites to give you the information whether you want to buy a dog that is certified to help someone with a hearing loss or you can take classes with your dog for your dog to be certified as a hearing dog. However, I had a professor in college who taught art history. She would bring yellow lab dogs throughout the semesters. She trained each dog and had that dog for a period of time until the dog was fully trained to be ready to go home to an owner. The dogs were polite and well trained. They would sit under the table while I sat in the front row. I gazed off to ponder my life or look at the dogs, wishing I could play with them! I had night classes; so on my way to the classes, I would see her teaching at least 15 people to train their labs to help people with deafness, blindness, or anything else. It is very common to see labs or golden retrievers helping people with needs; now it can be any breed as long as they are well trained and pass their courses.

Dogs who have been trained to respond to doorbells, phones ringing, even TDD, smoke detectors, babies crying, and alarm clocks going off. Also, they are trained to sit, heel, lie down, and come when you call them. While in training they are not allowed to be aggressive, sniff, beg, or jump on people. Finally they are trained to respond to things in the environment, like what you might encounter when out in the streets walking. Finally, they are trained to understand people who use sign language as communication; the dogs can understand the language and will do whatever their owner commands them to do. With all training they go through, it takes at least four to eight months to complete.

Who are qualified to have the hearing dogs? They must at least have 65 dB hearing loss, live alone or with others who are hearing, should not have any other dogs in the house, and can give the dog proper care. Also, they must be over eighteen years old to have a hearing dog that is certified. They have the right to bring their hearing dog anywhere as long as they have the ID card and the orange blaze collar on the dog. The public should not give them a hassle about bringing their dog. It is against the law. They can bring their dog on a bus or airplane when traveling, bring them to stores whether as grocery shopping or shopping for pleasure, and they can bring their dog to any appointments, such as to doctors. Basically, they are allowed to be anywhere with their owners. When going to places, people should not charge them an extra fee because they bring their dog with them. Even workplaces must allow them to bring their dog with them at all times, as it is allowed.

In a conclusion, I personally love dogs and strongly believe that they protect us and help us in the world when it comes to sounds in our environment that can make us feel secure in our own worlds. There are dogs that are specifically trained for deaf and blind people. I recommend getting one. You will not regret owning a dog! I think they bring the best out of our silent world. They definitely can make us feel loved and respected by them.

My Deaf Journey in Education and Social Life

I was born deaf. My parents did not realize it until I was at least ten months old when my brother suggested it to them that I might not hear right. He and I were playing around. He informed my mother, that as she called my name several times over and over to get my attention, I never responded to her. I would look up to her and smile while I continued to play. So my mother took me to a doctor in the town. Back in 1980s, he had pots and pans in his office. He banged them together by my ears. I was not supposed to see him doing that, but I have excellent eyesight. I saw him banging the pots together by my ears and successfully passed the tests. Then my mother brought me to an audiologist and several other doctors in their town. She got her answer that I was profoundly deaf.

Of course, my parents were devastated about it and did not know what to do from that point on. My mother took me to Clarke School for the Deaf in Boston. They, as well as other deaf schools had an oral program. She did her research. My parents brought me up oral and mainstreamed in public schools because they thought if I learned sign language at an early age, I would have a difficult time speaking with hearing people. They worried that if I learned sign language, as I get older, I might get lost somewhere and ask for help where people would not know how to communicate with me. At the time, we were living in Vermont, where my dad was running a flooring business next to our house. My mother would get calls from the elementary school down the road and was asked to come in for meetings.

I remember that during my preschool years I went to school and had a normal life as student. I had to wear my FM system in classes, where the teacher wore the microphone for my FM system. I had few teachers to work with for speech therapy. One woman, Sandy "Ba-Ba," definitely changed our lives. She would come and visit me at the house to teach me how to talk and reward me with candy to motivate me to speak. My mother would participate and get sick of eating peanut-butter candy as she would cringe as I forced her to eat it with me after we aced my speech lessons. Sandy also introduced me to another boy my age who needed help with speech therapy. He and I would spend time eating cake frosting and running around to play speech games. She was like a mother to me. I am almost 24 years old, and to our eyes she is part of the family. We meet her in Vermont every time we go back for a vacation.

While I was living back east I would spend every summer in Vermont, and she would take me out to the lake and historical places to teach me. Our relationship would be like Anne Sullivan and Helen Keller, where she worked very hard to help me with my speech, reading, and writing. While she was not with me for speech therapy, I had this guy who was my PE coach and speech therapist. For some reason, I was bored and angry with him. When I had to go to him for speech lessons, my father would trick me and tell me that we were going to the farm to get green beans or do strawberry picking. After a while he ran out of excuses to get me to go because I figured it all out. Finally, there was another woman who helped me during classes and in after-school daycare; I had to take a bus to a different part of town to go to this daycare center. This daycare center was for disabled kids, so I played with kids who were blind, in wheelchairs, and had learning disabilities. She would take care of me like as a babysitter on her days off.

School told my mother that I need to wear tee shirts and jeans more often than nice clothes, because I would roll down the hills of green grass and jump in the sandbox, as I thought it was rather exciting. I loved my nice clothes, and I refused to wear Wal-Mart clothes when I was only four years old. My mother and Sandy "Ba- Ba" had to go shopping together to get jeans and other clothes. Then school called again. My mother thought the call was about my clothes. Unfortunately, the call was not about my clothes; they wanted me to transfer to a deaf boarding school. My family decided it was time for a change, so my mother moved me and my brother to Beverly, Massachusetts, for a better program. The public school there had a specific program to help deaf children to be mainstreamed. We spent one hour with them for homework and catch up on our lessons in our classrooms. Jane and her sister Joan were in charge of the program, so I started working with them when I was in kindergarten.

One day after school I saw this girl drinking water out of the water fountain. Immediately, I saw her wearing hearing aids exactly like mine so I rushed down the hallway and grabbed her out of the water fountain area. I dragged her to my mother to inform her that she is just like me. My mother was just absolutely horrified for this girl, and she was not pleased with my shouting behavior with excitement. Ever since, she and I have been best friends. Ally and I would spend time together in the room with Jane and Joan. We would meet each other in the bathrooms as our classrooms were connected to each other with the bathroom. She was a year older; we would get caught by our teachers for meeting at places to hang out during the class time. I used to spend almost every weekend at her house if I was not going to Vermont to see my father with my family. I felt my life there was living out of a suitcase, because I either slept over at her house, visited my grandparents in Albany, New York, visited my father at our house in Vermont, or stayed at our house in Beverly, Massachusetts. Ally and I would take ice skating and gymnastics lessons together. I nicknamed us "The Keam Sisters," because when I was a little girl, I could not say, "ice cream." I said, "ice keam." So we took it from there. We would text each other our nickname to each other at the very end of our greetings. We fought over Zack on *Saved by the Bell,* as we had a crush on him when we were little girls. When we stayed past wee hours, we would get scared of the dark, so we kept the lights on and made up stories. At that time we had a code if we saw a ghost. We had to say, "Cheezits." For some reason, at that age, I already knew I was really different I wore hearing aids and had speech therapy when kids got out and played. The funny part is that while we were growing up, I would get frustrated with her because she would make me try to guess what songs she was humming from TV shows. I thought, *How can I guess if you are humming if we both are deaf?* Good times.

I had a normal childhood, but I worked hard because I had to go over homework and lessons all over again with my mother, as I did not get everything in the classroom, I had speech therapy, I went to Jane and Joan's for an hour a day to work on things to move ahead, and Joan sat next to me in the classrooms to assist me with work for most of the days. I continued to see my father in Vermont, as he was running the business and home, but my family decided it was time to move to Arizona after I completed 4th grade.

As you get older, peers expand and expand you develop a social life, fitting in groups and finding out who you are. I used to take ballet, hip hop, and jazz dance from the time I was four years old. I stopped taking the classes when I moved to Arizona, as it was a drastic change to adapt. I did not realize that when I got to a new school, they did not have a program like at the Cove School did for the almost five years I spent there. The kids in classes in Massachusetts were used to deaf kids because we had several in all grades over the years, so it seemed to me that they learned about our culture and who we are at a young age at the Cove School in Massachusetts. So then I went to this school Arizona school for a year. I was sure could not handle it anymore. I wanted to go back to Massachusetts to be able to fit in. The kids acted like we were very odd. My mother put me in a charter school in Scottsdale. The class size was from twelve to eighteen students. We had 5th and 6th grade classes combined together in a classroom. Also,

I met another deaf girl my age, but she had only a mild hearing loss. She and I went to school together for few years. She and I were a team together to gain respect from others. I had a lot of during those years, as we all became a family.

We left the charter school and went to a Christian school in Phoenix for a few years. We became cheerleaders and took state championship at the competitions. We also played girls basketball and volleyball. I did things that I would never imagine I would be able to do or get respect at doing. All the girls were very nice to us. The teachers made efforts to help us out. We had note takers in the classes we took. We did not wear FM systems, as the classrooms were small. There were times when a kid would ask me why I talked different from her; a lot of people cannot understand that the more hearing you have the better you can speak. The less hearing you have, the less you will speak like others. You might have a nasal tone or a slow talking rate. I had a teacher recommended me to go to a deaf school because of my speech and hearing loss; I was definitely devastated and had to face her for the rest of the spring.

Then going to high school, I was the only deaf student at my private Christian school going to this because of the area I lived in. I did not know anyone except my brother's friends, who were seniors. I did not have a boyfriend all through high school, as my brother told them that he would like them to watch out for me. They certainly did. Anyway, I had a few years when the only special resource for my disability was a teacher of the deaf that I met with for an hour every day at school. She helped me with classroom assistance by making sure my teachers met my IEP. My IEP said I had to have a note taker and sit up in the front of the classroom. Teachers must put closed captions on television when showing educational documentaries. I wasn't to have any oral quizzes, and teachers had to write notes on the board. I was behind again on reading and writing, so for four years of high school she helped me to master the level of reading and writing so that I was caught up with my class and prepared for college. At first I was frustrated with her, like Helen Keller was with Anne Sullivan, but I soon grew to love her and respect her for all the help she gave me, opening my eyes on the culture and my abilities in life.

I missed cheerleading, as I did it for few years during junior high, so I decided to try out for the junior varsity cheer squad at Chaparral High School. My mom hired a personal trainer to get me back in shape and work with me on my tumbling skills. He was a competition trainer for many squads. I knew him from previous years, as he helped us out in junior high where we took the state championship. I spent a few weeks working out with him every day for five hours, the maximum for these tryouts. I got to the gym. There were over 100 girls trying out for JV and varsity teams. I remembered just sitting on the floor in the gym with all the girls, all the girls hushed about me, trying out.

For a week, during classes and breaks, the girls spread rumors that I was trying out and not going to make it. My mother went to the coach of the teams; she informed my mother that they were just teenager girls with low self esteem, and that they were just saying things to scare me. She encouraged me to keep trying. I got to the tryouts and performed in front of seven judges that never knew any of us. I was tired and nervous. I was so sick after my tryouts that I did not go to school the next day. My mother and I went to school after the hours to see if my name was on the paper on the door. I had succeeded. We both cried. Of course, my mother decided to take me on a shopping spree to reward all the hard work I did.

I went back to school. Again there were rumors about how I made the cheerleading squad because I was deaf. What the school did not know was that the judges did not know I was deaf; it was not up to the coaches and former cheerleaders to pick. So I thought it was funny, and I continued to move forward with a uniform. I felt very good about myself when I cheered at all the games with the girls, did stunts and tumbling in front of the crowds, especially at pep rallies. People started to respect me better. I made the Varsity squad a year after, but we had a different coach, and she did not like my being deaf and performing with the girls. She clearly showed it to me and other girls in many ways, so I quit, and so did half of the squad due to their own personal reasons.

It is sad that kids at junior high school and high school can be cruel and don't know how to respect others and their backgrounds. I remember that my classmates would tease others whether they were overweight, short, and very tall, wearing glasses, kids who were disabled, anything. That's where insecurity or rebellion begins. Some kids who grew up secure changed in several ways, where their parents would look at their child wondering if it is just a phase or it is who they are. I watched students who had no manners to our teachers or the rest of us in the classrooms. I had a class in high school, video productions, where I was assigned to a partner. I found her to be outspoken and judgmental, as we spent time together working on projects to create videos that we would send out as daily news on TV, where seniors would do daily announcements along with all sorts of videos for a half hour. I always looked forward to that time of the day because I thought it was entertaining and different.

Anyway, she would make me feel like an idiot by not repeating things to me, or she would give me strange looks when we had conversations. She would always talk about herself. However, we kept interviewing people around the campus. My teacher thought we should do things evenly, but she ended up always interviewing people while I would videotape. I soon came to realized that I always videotaped the interviews, so I told her that I had to interview people as well, because our teacher wanted us to work as a team and do things evenly. She refused. Then she directly told me that I could not interview the students on campus because of my terrible speech. I asked her what did she specifically mean by that? She answers that I should not be talking at all, I did not belong at the school, and my speech was not good enough for the video. I felt sad at the moment. I told her she had no right to talk to me that way where she had an absolute no idea where I came from and how hard I worked to work with my hearing loss and speech. After that, I walked up to my teacher and told her what happened. She let me work on my own projects after that.

After graduating from high school, I went to Scottsdale Community College for a semester. I felt like I was going to a high-school reunion every day because so many of my classmates were all over the campus at college. I struggled a little bit at first with classes and soon, I decided it was time for me to leave the town for a while. I was going through a difficult time with family and friends, so I moved to Los Angeles to live with my uncle. He helped me to boost my confidence level. He taught me to shake hands firmly with others, because it shows them I am confident. We learned about each other, as we were different. It was a great time to learn something valuable, and I am sure I taught him few things in life as well. I realized I had been sheltered by my family and group of best friends. When I got to Los Angeles, here I was driving myself around the crazy freeways, going to the beach alone, buying my very first newspaper, first toothbrush, doing a lot of things by myself. I soon became very independent; I met new people through my uncle, as we were at least 18 years apart, so he took me out.

Over the summer I drove to Kernville, California, a couple of times to visit my best friend, Brooke, from high school. She was working at a rafting company for the summer. I met people who were respectful and used sign language because there was a girl who I became very close with, Kate. She is deaf; her communication is sign language and oral. She introduced me to another side of the silent world. I fell in love with sign language; I found it easy to communicate without a struggle, since it was visual language for me. All the rafting guides who learned sign language through her were signing with me, and there I was, deaf all my life, and I did not know any signs, so I chose to study the culture and learn sign language for two years in college when I returned after that summer. I went back to Scottsdale Community College for a few semesters; I was getting help from the Disability Resource Center, where I was receiving help from the note takers in classes.

After studying arts and sign language for a year and half, I transferred to Paradise Valley Community College to take biology class with John and his cousin. I had to start all over again, getting help to transfer my disability paperwork. The first month was extremely difficult, as biology was my weak subject. My professor was a very kind man; he lectured for two to five hours, two days a week, and the tests were out of his lectures and rarely out of the book. So I failed my first test where I studied for days trying to pass the test. In the meantime, I went back and forth with Disability Resource Center to get the right kind of help. At first they gave me a tape recorder, which I thought was strange! So the other option they gave me was a video camera recorder. They set it up in the back of the classroom, and you can see my professor roaming around the classroom, writing on several different boards around the room. I watch television with closed captions, so I informed them that the tapes were not working for me. I felt I was trying to find Waldo in the tapes because it was too far away for me to lip read him! Finally, after a month of going through this, they hired a woman to type lectures on the computer in the classroom. I finally felt I belonged in the classroom and watched what she typed; I did not feel like I was left out. I started acing my tests shortly after that; it made a *huge* difference! She typed what he was saying. It felt like I was reading closed captions in the classroom. I watched the screen while she was typing what he was saying. Then she would email it to me after she revised it for a few hours shortly after the class. I would print it out and put it in my notebook; I studied and looked in the lectures for answers for the study guides he gave us. I started out with an "F" and ended with an "A."

I remember that difficult teachers I have had would make me cry because they would use their own materials to teach; I would find it difficult to learn with my deafness. Also, I would study and study with my mother or friends for a week for an important exam; I would fail it because I would not understand what the question was asking exactly, that made it harder for me to answer it correctly. Looking back, I can see a few professors in my mind yelling at me and telling me that I did not study at all. I cried in front of them. I even scared them off. They were males. Go figure! Clearly I can see the memories, and me talking to one college professor. He who was really intelligent and excellent at teaching us all sorts of arts; he was like our drill sergeant only because he wanted us to learn and see what he was seeing. I cried to him, saying I was really trying hard; I had a lot of stuff going on my plate, such as taking care of my grandmother and the rest of family with health problems to help my mother out. He was appalled and backed off; he began to help me even more through the lessons with patience and respect. I enjoyed everything he taught me, no matter if he had to repeat teaching me until I got it.

"You can't always sit in your corner of forest and wait for people to come up to you. You have to go to them sometimes." Winnie the Pooh

Classroom Accommodations

Wondering how to teach a deaf student, how your child learns in the classroom, or even wonder how to learn with all the help you can get from Disability Resource Center? There are several ways of learning with all types of assistance to pave the way for you to learn. The technology and ways of helping children and young adults are growing as people find ways to meet our needs over the years. I cannot wait to see what the future has to offer for educating our children with needs!

Notetaker:

There are few ways to find a note taker for you in the class. First the teacher can pick out a student that has excellent grades in the class and see if you want that person to be your note taker for the class. Then you and the teacher ask the student. Mostly they say yes. It is normal if they act nervous and feel like they have a responsibility for your grades. Just comfort them and compliment their notes. Another way is teachers will announce in class that they need a student to volunteer to write notes for you. After classes you will find someone who comes up with an interest in helping you as a note taker. Remember the teacher does not have the right to announce your name unless you give them your permission to say so. Then the Disability Resource Center might need the note taker's name and information, like they did in college with mine. They always provide you and your note taker a non- carbon replicating (NCR) notepaper. When the notetaker writes notes on this, the notes will also show up on the piece of paper below, which saves you both time from copying paper at a copy machine, and you two each have your own notes for your binders.

Front Row Seating:
The teacher and Disability Resource Center will recommend a deaf student to sit up in the front row of the classrooms if being mainstreamed at a school. This way the deaf student can understand what the teacher is saying by lip reading and hearing them closer instead of sitting in the back row where you see heads in front of you and cannot hear as much as the people who sit up in the front row. There should be no struggle to write notes down, as the people might have in the back row shifting their bodies' right to left to see what to write from the board. I have sat up in the front row in my life in all schools I went to. I hated it because my good friends would be in the back, or people would chat back and forth in the back while I sat up in the front with nothing going on. At least I was understanding what was going on and getting the right kind of help. Also, I could not be normal like other students. I could not pass notes, talk across the room for friends to lip read me and my facial expressions, because the teachers always made sure I was learning and understanding their teaching methods. I know they did their best and really wanted me to learn more than any other students as they did not want to see me struggle.

Guidelines Typed:
Teachers have guidelines to teach students that they print it out for deaf students to follow their instructions as the teachers read them out loud. Also, they type it on the overhead projector or Power Point Presentation as short notes and outlines for study guides. I had a fantastic English Teacher at Chapparal High School for three years; he learned how to help me out while teaching, and he did one of these methods. He did an assignment on *Romeo and Juliet* among other novels on Power Point Presentation with questions, answers, and

theories. He even printed the information for me, so I could take it home and study it.

Computer Aide Note Taker:
The Disability Resource Center hires a person to be transcriptionist for a deaf student where they type lecture notes on the computer while the student reads it. They normally sit next to each other. Sometimes if this seating can't be worked out, the deaf student will read it on her computer while the transcriptionist is typing on her own laptop somewhere else in the room.

I only had transcriptionists, two different women for different classes in college. One woman would revise her notes and e-mail them to me right away after class. We would use the classroom printers, or she would e-mail it to me at home, and I would print it to put it in my notebook for study materials. The other one only printed it right after the class; they all used spell check on Microsoft Word so it sped up the time to revise their notes.

Sign Language Interpreters:
The Disability Resource Center provides a sign language interpreter for deaf students who use ASL as their communication. The interpreter sits next to or in front of the student in the classroom. They only sign what the teacher and students say orally. They normally cannot participate to help you with your assignments when the students have to ask others questions like the teacher does or students if they are doing a group project.

Personal Assistant/ Oral Interpreter:
Again, this is very similar to a sign language interpreter, except they do not use sign language. They assist the students making sure they are following the instructions and being on the same page with others. Also, they would talk to the students about what the teacher said for clarification or repeat what the teacher said if the student gets puzzled.

I had one when I was in grade school who helped me to do the assignments on time with other students, like projects, quizzes, and readings. She would tell me what was going on most of the time. She would not tell me the answers or how to do it, like she would not do the work for me. She would assist me step by step as the teachers gave instructions to us in the classroom.

Closed Captioned Video on TV:
Teachers should always put closed caption on TV for deaf students to be part of the learning environment. If the video does not have closed caption on it, they should order those that do through websites that the Disability Resource Center will provide for you. In high school, there were VHS tapes that were older and did not provide closed captioning, so my teacher of the deaf would order the film to rent off the website, so I could watch it in the class. When I was in college, in biology class we did not have a TV; we had a projector, so it did not provide closed captioning. However, my professor would let me rent videos out of the library ahead of time and watch it at home with closed captioning so I could write answers and essay questions on time in class.

My Experiences Dating in the Silent World

While I was growing up and going to several different schools, there were always boys and girls liking each other in classes while being shy and coy with each other. Those were days when we experienced crushes, school relationships where we didn't see our boyfriends/girlfriends after school all the time if we were in 3rd grade and lived far from each other. There were dances or cute Valentine's cards with a piece of candy that we had to bring to the elementary school that we went to. Sometimes things are embarrassing, crushing hurtfully, or if we are lucky, we have something that we will cherish that gives us a reason to keep believing in love. I consider myself unlucky due to my low self esteem while growing up, but I would consider myself lucky that there were few guys who respected me, and I am still friends with them to this day.

First, before I go on and sharing my stories about boys, another thing that brought down my self esteem was my image. My image? Poor me. I had hearing aids that looked like a walkman player early in the days. I wore glasses with a patch on one of eyes. I was a little chubby—I am trying not to be cruel to myself! Also, I wore retainers, then braces at the age of ten years old. I had to wear night head gear in bed. I was already a "woman" by that time. I swear, my family, even my dad's side of the family, thought of me when they saw the movie, *Little Miss Sunshine,* as the little girl with glasses who wanted to be in the beauty pageant. I was very much like her. They also thought, what else could I possibly go through, as I looked like a child trying to balance myself with all these things on me! I felt very unattractive when I was a little girl. So I told myself not to focus on wanting a boyfriend where I wanted to focus on my education and have friends along with freedom.

I had few crushes while growing up. My brother always had friends over playing with us while we played hide and seek in the dark at the warehouse around the carpets every summer after playing basketball. I felt normal. I felt confident because they accepted me and included me. Of course, I had crushes on his friends. I did not realize who I was as a deaf person, and how kids at my own age, especially boys, can be immature and worry about their image when I was in middle school and high school. For them it was all about being popular or their reputation.

When I started junior high at a new school I felt very self conscious about my deafness. People did not know for a while that my friend and I were deaf, as we kept it to ourselves and tried to lead a normal life there as much as we could. It was a hard stage, where we wanted to be accepted and do not know how much they would understand about our deafness. We got closer with the girls after few weeks; they figured out that we're deaf. The boys had not really figured it out by then. So one day, a girl told them, because she found out that there were few boys that liked us. I was sad because the boys acted weird around us. I cried on the way home to my house. I felt very uncomfortable with myself, as I thought I would not be loved by a man someday. My parents told me that they were not worth my tears if they treated me like that way.

I continued to go to school, and I did not really pay any attention to them, while things were awkward for a while. During that time, I developed a wonderful friendship with a boy. We hung out all the time at school, met out at the mall with friends and were really together all the time on field trips to California or other places. He was really caring to me and the best friend you could ask for. I remember that we got in trouble one day because the boys pushed us into the bathroom. As he took something from me, like a hair clip, on the way out of the bathroom, there was our principal behind me. He was 6 feet

5 inches tall or so. We were in trouble. Anyway, this friend of mine never betrayed me, he respected my deafness, and he cared for me. We developed a crush on each other; one day I thought he asked me to kiss him at the school in front of everyone. I freaked out, and he joked and said, "Here is the kiss." It was a Hershey's kiss. Everyone thought we were going to end up together after we graduated from middle school. We went to a few high school dances together, as we went to different schools. We saw other people some over the past few years, so he always tells me that if we are single when we are 25 or older, we will just get married, because we are best friends. So we remain as close friends to this day. Although our lives are different now, he and I keep in touch often.

At the same time, I was dealing with boys at my high school. I remember being a new girl at the school, and after a month went by, I saw boys just telling their friends that I was deaf. One day, I really got fed up with this group of older guys. They said something to each other about me and did not think I was able to catch what they said. So I went up to them and told them that I saw what they said about me.

They asked, how did I know?

I told them, "I can lip read very well."

Instantly, they were really red and felt embarrassed. So few days later a guy asked me out in the hallway, and I told him no because of what they said previously. Later on my friends and I went to the football games to support our high-school football team. I had met few guys there during the season, and we exchanged screen names, as they were students at different schools. I told them that I was deaf and could not talk on the phone. They were okay with that. I did not think anything would happen after that, especially with my cochlear implant surgery coming up. A month went by. I was asked out on dates by few different guys. My brother did not like it that they were seniors, as I was freshman, and that they drove me on dates. I remembered he was yelling at my parents in their bedroom for letting me go on a date, as my date could hear him. I was horrified. I was really stressed out with my cochlear implant recovery and adjusting to sounds, and I had cheerleading tryouts coming up, so I took a break from boys.

During my sophomore year I met a few guys who became my best friends. To this day we still see each other every once in a while. One friend he was in my math class, and I did not know it until he talked to me a few times; he asked me to be his Valentine. I freaked out, as I was still incredibly shy and did not want to deal with dating, as I was on the cheer team going to practices every morning before school and after school, then games. He still gave me Valentine stuff after I told him no and why. He asked me out several times throughout the years. I just felt he was my best friend, and I did not want to change a thing there. He even took me to his family's charity ball. I was wearing his father's jewelry, and I had bodyguards around us. He didn't see my deafness as anything; he treated me as "Ashlee." I had another few guy friends who were close with us in the group; of course there was a lot of drama because of crushes here and there. I was still shy and did not want to get my hopes up getting my first boyfriend if the drama was going to ruin it.

One summer my family and I went to the beach in California for a week. As my parents and I were walking to the beach, a boy waved at me and ran up to his balcony to watch me swim out in the ocean. Somehow my family and I hung out with him and his family during that week. We ran into them on the pier. I told my parents not to tell him I was deaf because of my personal experiences from school, so he thought I was just shy. Few days later, my father and I were out swimming and boogie boarding the waves. He and his cousins came out with us; we told him that I was deaf, as I could not hear a thing out in the water. He was fine with it; we played volleyball games with his family and watched movies with our families. We still keep in touch to this day.

I figured my life out with guys and moved on. I moved to California to figure out who I was and get out of my shell. I stayed in Los Angeles for at least six months. I stayed in Kernville for the summer, well, actually, two summers in a row. I had older guys take me out. I realized that they did not care. They actually thought I was attractive just because I was confident and open about my deafness. Most of all, I stood out, as I am different from others. I have stories to tell. I was able to socialize with them and their friends. I realized that I went through an awkward teen phase that we all go through, because the older I get, I continue to meet adults who are mature and do respect me for who I am. I started to see myself in a different way. I felt more confident. From that point on, I really tell the guys that I am deaf. Even when my close friend is from South Africa and she has an accent, they would ask me where I was from. I told them about my deafness; they actually thought I was from London or Switzerland. I took it as a compliment at the time, hah! I remembered Kate and I met a guy at a pool-hall bar. He asked us questions, so we told him that we were deaf. He was not really aware of what deaf is really about, so he asked us several questions. It was a weird moment.

Now I look at girls who I know are deaf; they are in their 20s, and they don't really tell guys that they are deaf right away because of fears for getting rejected. I noticed how, if we notify them immediately and act confident, they love girls with good self esteem. They do not want to deal with girls who have low self esteem. If we girls get rejected or mistreated by guys, it is not worth our tears and our time! We shall not let them affect our self esteem. I realized that if you don't love yourself, you will have a hard time with life and finding love because the person will have a hard time figuring out how to fall in love with you. Robert Frost once said "Don't ever take a fence down until you know why it was put up," where it seems to me that if you do not accept yourself, learn to accept who you are, and let the walls down to start exploring who you are and accept the opportunities awaiting for you.

Soon I figured the guys I liked, and it did not work out, because "The One" is on his way to me battling through the jungle to complete my heart. If girls use guys to be in relationships because they are afraid of being alone, it is going to take them a long time to find the right one. I realized that being deaf is absolutely not a bad thing after all! Because I tend to be different from others, this is the main quality about me that strikes everyone else out there. I am far different from them and stand out. I have stories to tell to people; my life is interesting, so I can teach someone a lesson or two about being different and accepting yourself. I like this quote by e. e. Cummings: "It takes courage to grow up and become who you really are."

Finally one night I informed my family that I was not going to get a boyfriend because I loved my single life and did not want to deal with the drama. The following night, I went to Brooke's house to hang out; she had her neighbors over at her house, as they were close to our age. She warned me about the boys before I got to meet John. I thought it was strange of her to say that because she never did that before, and we always talk about how we did not want to be in relationships all the time. So I told her I did not care because I was not looking for anything. I met John and his brother, Lee. At first, I thought John was annoying because he was throwing the dogs' toys, such as balls around me and Brooke as she and I were signing to each other. I did not find out till later on that he was doing that to get my attention, as he thought I was attractive. So we all decided to go to the batting cage. I seriously did not think he liked me at the moment. We all went up for a drive up to the mountains to see the city lights. I remembered just thinking in the car on the way up there that he was different; there was something about him, and I wanted to get to know this guy. I don't know why, but I did feel something there while I was looking at the stars during the drive. As we all got out looking at the stars and city lights, he brought the blanket and wrapped me up in his arms with the blanket. I normally would get nervous about this, but I did not. I could feel his heart beating fast. We got back to Brooke's house; we exchanged numbers, as I told him I do not talk on the phone. He texted me on my way home to my parents. We went to see a movie the following night and hung out every night for two weeks. Then it was time for Brooke and my move to California for the summer for our rafting jobs.

So over the summer I told him that we needed time apart, not chatting on AIM or texting. He was going to visit, but I wanted to enjoy my summer there with my friends. I worked long hours almost every day, so I did not want to ruin our thing that we had. When I returned, he treated me with a dinner and asked me to be his girlfriend. I told him I needed time to think about it. He told all his friends that we were already a couple, so I gave in and said yes. I was worried only just because I had never been in relationship before, so I was concerned that he might not have enough patience with my deafness. Soon he showed me he did by printing papers about deaf culture, sign language, cochlear implants and other types of deaf research to show that he was interested in me and my deafness. He would always put closed caption on TV or movies to make sure I was able to understand everything. He would serenade songs to me as he would sing along to the words as I could not hear the lyrics. When we went out with our friends whether I was hanging out with his or mine, he would tell me what they said or why they laughed if I looked lost. I was impressed because I never had to ask him why they were laughing or to repeat what they said. We ended up taking biology class together; he ended up being an amazing supporter when I was going through a difficult time trying to get help from Disability Resource Center for that class. While I was waiting for the right kind of help, he translated what our professor said to me while he helped me study for our exams.

One evening he took me out for a dinner at PF Chang's. As we were finishing up with our three-course meals our fortune cookies came. He took his fortune cookie immediately. I really am particular about picking mine, but he did not let me pick, so I thought that was strange at the moment. So I opened mine. I actually did not read the whole thing. I saw that it said, "Ashlee Rose…." Then I stopped and looked at the ceiling because I was amazed that the fortune cookie had my name in it. I was in a "wow" moment. So I went back to read the rest of it. It said, "Ashlee Rose, will you marry me?" I was absolutely in shock! Of course, I said yes. I thought it was a perfect way to propose because it was visual for my deafness. It was beyond incredibly romantic to me. So we celebrated with our families at my parents' house with dessert and drinks. We did break up for a few days, as we realized a lot of things, but we got back together by not letting others control our relationship and we wanted to start a journey together. There were families who were worried about our relationship, as we were young, and they were concerned about my being a deaf wife and deaf mother. Now, we have a baby girl, and he is totally supportive of and unconcerned about my being a deaf mother. I am lucky for that. We have worked extremely hard on our personal issues and with our situation as deaf and hearing. It works for us. I always enjoy our relationship. I feel we are a good match: he wears glasses, and I wear hearing aids, so by the end of the night, we would put them on the dresser, and I would tease how that is when we enter being deaf-and-blind couple. I even saw a tee shirt at a store with three monkeys: "I see no evil," "I hear no evil," and "I speak no evil." John would see no evil, I hear no evil, and our daughter (should) speak no evil!

It is not that I did not want to date or marry a deaf man; I actually have never had a relationship with them. Just the way my life took me on this path, I ended up in the oral hearing world with relationships with people such as John. There are times I have asked myself, would I date a deaf man? I have thought it would be a lot of work because of getting their attention or dealing with our situations related to deafness, but at the same time I looked at it as it could be less work where we would have to be patient with each other, as we both would know what it is like to be deaf. I know deaf people feel it is not an issue, but do want to explore the hearing world for their personal reasons while the rest are married to their deaf partner. We are entitled to be with who we want to be; no one can stop or tell us who we should be. We need to know the value of love by listening to our hearts. We have the power over who we want to love and be loved by.

In this world there are several categories where people are diverse, such as in race, money, sexuality, and disabilities. For an example, in the movie, *Titanic*, Rose was in love with a poor man, Jack, but her parents did not approve of him. She went ahead and listened to her heart as he showed her how to trust and believe in life. The same thing happened with the film, *the Notebook*, where Allie fell in love with a man that her parents did not approve of. Noah and Allie fought their way back to each other, as they found it was true love. Every day there is someone being in love with someone who is different from them or who has a different lifestyle. It is just up to them, as "Love conquers all." I took few courses in sociology at Scottsdale Community College about marriage and personal relationships. I learned a lot and found it interesting how we all learn who we are as individuals. I learned that relationships hold a strong bond through trust where people put their walls down. They should work on their personal problems to get rid of their baggage in their relationship. As different cultures can form together as a team, couples learn how to compromise and respect their cultures. They must be committed as a family or a couple to work on their relationship daily to show affection and support.

Being a Parent of a Deaf Child and Being a Deaf Parent of a Hearing Child

Wondering how to provide a life for your child when he or she is born, having dreams for your child that you hope your child has a better life than what you had, and pondering about what to do with a child of yours who is deaf? I am a deaf child of my parents; I do not understand what parents go through when they find out their child is deaf. My parents and the rest of my family would exchange stories about how they felt when they first found out about my deafness. I listened to them as I understood about myself, but I would never understand what my parents had to go through in their commitment to get me to where I am today, because I will never be able to be in their shoes since I am already deaf. However, I am a deaf mother to my hearing daughter. She is already few months old, so I am still learning about being a deaf mother to her.

How to start with what to do with your child who is deaf? You can start out with goals depending on education, technology, and what your community offers. First, you should do your personal research for what your community and the state that you live in offer to help you with your child. Second, you can interview people like audiologists and doctors for what they do with deaf children. They can give you suggestions. Third, you should go to schools where deaf children go, such as deaf school, and where they go to public schools to be mainstreamed so you can watch how the kids socialize with each other and how the teachers teach their students. Ask around the campus if there are parents there or ask the administration for more information.

You should see a difference in social life and education for your child at the deaf schools and public schools. If you know people who are dealing with a similar situation to yours, ask them what their personal experiences are.

Education is very important. For your child to pass each grade and move forward seems like an American dream to all families. Public schools have programs like Disability Resource Centers. When I went to elementary school there was only one department that specialized in assisting deaf children with classrooms, technology, homework, class work, and speech therapy. Find out what they do exactly—whether they teach in groups with other kids or provide alone time with your child to do all the work you would like to see your child do. Sometimes, education that offers the most for your child is not in your community. It requires moving the family to a town that provides everything you need for your child. My mother moved my brother and me to Massachusetts from Vermont for me to get help.

Perhaps you should think about what would work for you and your family with your child. Do you want your child to speak or use sign language? If your child is an infant, you would have to make decisions, but if your child is old enough to understand, your child has a right to make decisions as well. Remember to talk to your partner first, as marriage is a commitment, to remain healthy you and your spouse must work together to figure out what to do with a child who is deaf. You shall understand the commitment in teaching your child to communicate because you would have to provide speech therapy or lessons for your child to learn sign language. If your child learns sign language, the rest of your family should join in as well so they can all be able to communicate and play with your child. I met deaf people who learned sign language later on and use it as communication, but very few of their family members know sign language, so they cannot communicate with the rest who do not know the language. Learning the language is dependent upon time management. It is important to participate because it is a bond between your child and the family to share the love and be on a journey together.

Hearing all sounds that your child can respond to comes through a hearing aid or cochlear implant. Technology is advancing and growing rapidly to be used for comfort and security. If you want your child to grow up oral, be mainstreamed at school, and have every opportunity you can dream of, these devices would be recommended. However, I would not specifically recommend which is the best for your child, since I have experienced several devices during my deaf journey. My situation just happens to fall in place with the way it started out to where I am now. I have opened my eyes and learned more about the other side of the deaf culture where not all of them wear hearing aids or have a cochlear implant. I have a few friends that wear one hearing aid and others do not wear a hearing aid at all, as they feel comfortable about themselves and their culture. Think about the environment you wish your child to be in. Ask around to find out what kind of lifestyle your child is going to have. If you live in a busy city, maybe you should. If you live in a small town, maybe you don't have to. I remembered the deaf school in Phoenix a year ago was having a talk about how students should wear at least a hearing aid in the classrooms. So I recommend you to do your investigation, you will feel better as you gather your questions and answers together. The only warning I will give out is that there will always be people telling you what they think you should do. Be prepared; it may seem like they are pushing you as they are giving their opinions to you. All people are entitled to have their opinions, but they do not get to make the decisions for you. You and your partner are the first priority to make decisions and ask your children if they are old enough to understand.

Making a decision can seem to be overwhelming for you to decide; you can always change your mind and change plans at any time. This is not a permanent decision that you will have to make. It can change everyone's life, but it is not the most tragic thing that ever happened to you. If your child decides that he or she wants to go to a deaf school later on instead of public school and be oral, you should support that decision entirely. My parents would be sad for me if I come home crying from a difficult day about my hearing impairment. My parents would tell me that they wished they could be in my silent shoes for the day to know what it is exactly like to be deaf and what it feels like to go through. Like I said earlier, we cannot be in your shoes, and you cannot be in our shoes to understand, but we can listen to each others' souls.

My mother loved the song, "What a Wonderful World," by Louie Armstrong because we went to Florida for a deaf convention, as she wanted to seek more information about parenting and how to provide a life for your child who is deaf. At the end the people who hosted it enclosed pictures of me and rest of the other deaf children there as a slide show, along with the song, "What a Wonderful World." She cried and fell in love with it. I will never understand what my mother went through to raise a deaf daughter. There were times when we would argue, and she would cry, telling me I have no idea how much she had done for me. Being a parent is a joyful thing but it is yet a difficult thing to do to raise children in their own environment.

My family has been amazing to me since I was born deaf. They accepted me and tried to give me as normal a life as they could offer. My mother had a lot of patience with me. She cleaned teeth all day and picked me up at the daycare center; then we would go home, and she would teach me what my teachers taught on that day. Then we would do homework together. When we would finish up my homework we'd start our speech-therapy lessons. She was my best friend ever since I was born. I remember when I was five years old telling my mother she had to come live with me when I went to college because I was that attached to her. She would take me to work with her if I was sick, as she had no babysitter available for me and was running late. I enjoyed going to her work and watching her clean people's teeth. I colored my coloring books while I was close with the secretary in Massachusetts, where she fed me a lot of M&Ms. I remember my mother asked me on the way to work when I was sick if I was happy that I did not have to go to school and go to spend time with her. She told me that I did not look sick.

I responded to her, "Mom, I am sick. It is not out here, I hurt in here, so I do not look like I am sick."

My father has been my coach as he supported me when I wanted to play basketball or do some modeling, as he is a photographer. He would know something was wrong with me if I tried to act like nothing happened, and I would cry when he said, "What is wrong?" He goofed around and played pranks on all of us, as I remembered he put a dead lizard on my pillow. My dog was sniffing my face, and I wondered why my face was wet and smelly. He had found a bloated dead lizard out in the pool in our backyard. I made him sleep in my bed for three nights because I was horrified. My brother and I protected each other when we grew up as we moved around together and experienced a lot of personal crises we had in our family. He would include me playing with his friends. Even when he was in high school, I would go out with him and his friends to play basketball or to a haunted house. He really took care of me while we played pranks on each other or fought against each other even though we love each other.

On a sunny Sunday afternoon where the weather was perfect in Arizona in April, it was very cool. Although the perfect sun warmed us in the desert, at night it got chilly. I was out shopping with John and my mother at Costco's as we were getting food for my grandmother, and at the time, I was nine months pregnant, waiting to deliver my daughter. We moved in her home few weeks before my daughter arrived so I could take care of my grandmother who has Alzhiemer's. My whole life, she has been so good to my family, and she is my best friend. Sadly, she was diagnosed with Alzheimer's a few years ago. I have taken care of her on and off for the last five years. This time, we decided to move in while John worked for an electrical company. That way I could be her care giver and be at home being a mother to my daughter. However, I thought I must be really out of shape on this day when we were walking around the store. I was not aware of my contractions, as I had been nesting like crazy! Anyway, we got back and I complained to John about my back pains and the rest of my symptoms. He called the doctor; my doctor said it was time to come in.

I thought it was perfect because I had just met my doctor on Friday afternoon with my mother. John and I had just moved from Tucson, so I had had to find a new doctor. I enjoyed meeting him; he told me that my water could break any time till my due date, which was two weeks after that day I met him. He informed us that he was on schedule to work over the weekend but was off on Monday. For some reason, I told John that I was not going to the hospital because I did not want it to be false alarm then come back home. Everyone thought I was crazy. My parents came to the house and said it was time to go, so we went to the hospital. As we walked in the lobby, my water definitely broke. I could not believe it happened in the lobby out of everywhere. What good timing! Wow. So we checked in. I felt good just experiencing back labor. The nurse gave me antibiotics in my arm with an IV. I seriously asked John and the nurse if it was normal to have contraction in my arm!

Because I was experiencing pains due to the high dosage of meds in my arm, I was scared every time they refilled it. I thought I was going to be fine but after six hours went by she was still not ready to arrive. I started thinking about my being a deaf mother. *Was she going to be deaf or hearing? The labor was going to be painful, and more.* I started crying in the bathroom with my mother and Brooke. I told them I did not want it to come out of me because I was scared it was going to hurt badly. They laughed and comforted me. Then another eight hours went by. I needed epidural and could not receive it right away because I was not ready, and I told them I needed it and I am definitely ready! I cried again to everyone in the room, being all nervous about the procedure of delivering my daughter.

I had watched a lot of documentaries over the winter time on delivering babies; they showed that there were a lot of nurses and doctors pulling the babies out. I thought, *What if I mess up or don't do what they want me to when I do not understand them?* John assured me that he would repeat what the doctor said. I grabbed John and told him I was going to kill him. That was how much pain I was in! He always talked about this particular moment, one of his favorite moments. Finally at noon time on Monday it was time to slowly push. It was just me and John with the nurse. She was absolutely wonderful to us. I thought how it was not stressful and how peaceful my environment was at the moment because it was quiet. Then my doctor came in even on his time off. He did not want me to go through meeting yet a third doctor, so he saved me from a lot of stress off. My daughter was born. She had a lot of dark hair. On my family's side, we all were blondes and bald, while those on John's side were brunette and had a lot of hair.

I was puzzled by the beauty of my daughter. I heard her cry; I watched her mouth rolling her tongue as if she was trying to do some Spanish speaking in a crying tone. I cried at how I finally did it. I had overcome my fears. Everyone went home except John, who stayed with me at the hospital for four days. The first night I was scared and literally exhausted. I was scared because I have never taken care of a baby before, and I didn't know how to feed her, how often she was going to wake us up, was she going to be a crying baby, and more thoughts traveled on. I had several nurses that came in on their shifts. I would inform them right away that I was deaf and needed help. They took good care of me. I remembered I did not sleep very much when John was sleeping, as when he was out, he did not hear our daughter cry much because we were exhausted. So I was concerned and took little naps and kept peeking over by my bed to look at her. Then I would get the butterflies feeling in my stomach, thinking, *She is real, she is mine, and what a beauty she is!* We were anxious to go home, itching to start our lives immediately as a family. She barely cries even to this day. She is already a few months old and is a very easy baby to take care of.

As you all know I am deaf, and I am a mother of my daughter who is a few months old. Of course I am scared. These are my thoughts: *will my daughter ever understand who I am, how I am deaf, why I talk like this? Will she ever understand when I talk? Will she respect me for who I am and love me, How do I explain to her about me and how to communicate with me? I have a hard time understanding toddlers when they are learning how to talk, how will I understand my own child who is asking me to give her food or she is tired?*

Everyone I know worries that I will not be able to hear my baby cry or calling me. They worry about my being a deaf mother, especially me being in a relationship with a hearing man. They fear that he would have no patience and walk out on me and my daughter because my deafness could add more work for him, as he can hear our daughter crying at 3 o'clock in the morning while I am sound asleep. I feel nobody knows how to be a parent until they begin their parenting by bringing their own child into this world, so I am not going to know everything about being a mother, since my daughter is only a few months old. I absolutely love her! All I know is that John and I have a routine on parenting along with my deafness, where he helps me out, while I help him out. We continue to learn our roles.

During my pregnancy I did not know if our daughter was going to be deaf or hearing. I did not know you can go and get tested if you and your partner are committing to it, where the results are taken afterwards. I know someone who is deaf, and so is her husband. They already knew their son was deaf when she was pregnant with him because they took tests. I think it is amazing to be able to know already whether your child is deaf or not. I have not taken it nor any other tests that they offer. John and I thought we would just take one day at a time and embrace the birth of our daughter and take care of stuff afterwards.

After researching several websites about deaf parents of a hearing child, it seemed to be a positive experience, because the deaf parents can show their children what their culture is about. I have read that there are camps, picnics, and other events where the groups of deaf parents meet, with their hearing kids, to socialize. To me it shows that the kids will have a better understanding of who we are, and can play with other hearing kids who have a deaf parent, and see that that is normal. It will give them a better sense of their foundation and culture. Also, I think the kids will respect us and our needs, such as communicating with us properly by watching our kids expressing their own feelings. The stories I have read about parenting hearing babies, they never leave the room until they have another adult in charge, so they can take a shower or cook dinner. They have assisted-living devices and hearing dogs that notify them if anything arises with their hearing child.

I do not have the equipment yet that alerts me when the baby cries. I do not have the money for the stuff out there that the parents are able to buy for their nursery room. I had help from others. My uncle is in process of helping me with my deaf needs for my daughter's care, as I am taking care of his mother at the same time. For now, John wakes me up to let me know that she is crying, and I will get up and feed her bottle every night. He was out of town for almost a month for electrical work; I was on my own to take care of my daughter and my grandmother. I am doing a routine where I keep her awake until 2 a.m. then I would wait for her to wake up, and then feed her. After that, I would go to sleep with her as she lay in bed with me and kicked me in the mornings when she woke up. She is definitely mommy's alarm clock lately!

I have realized that I will be the best mother I can be by finding ways to be there for my daughter through technology and the system that John and I continue to work on, especially around our families. I am always around my daughter, as I am a care giver and stay-at-home mother. I show her all the love I have because I need to make sure she is okay and happy at all times. I want her to know that we love her. Also, I have overcome several obstacles in my life with my deafness, where I feel at this moment, I can conquer my fears about being a deaf mother of a hearing child and be the best person I can be for my small family. Even though I failed at a lot of things in life, or have been put in a difficult situation against my deafness, I had several opportunities to face it until I succeed at it. This taught me what my strengths are, along with teaching patience skills.

While my daughter grows up I am going to be a role model to her and remind her not to give up at things, because I have not, and look at where I am in life today. I have looked around and realized that many people who are disabled or have a problem, they continued on with their parenting skills. Heather Whitestone and Marlee Matlin both have children and seem to be happy with their family lives. Christopher Reeves I have always admired with my heart while I was growing up. He continued being a husband and father to his own family while he was in his wheelchair. Often I saw him on the news. His smile was like sunlight rays with a great spirit and happiness because he and his family loved each other, and they worked things out.

No matter what our cases are, we can continue to live a normal life in this world and have normal things, such as marriage and family. Even the roles of being married or parents, we choose to be on the path because we want to take the responsibility for it or we want to expand the chart level of "love and nurture." I may be deaf, but my eyes and my heart are not deafened. I have as big a soul as you will ever meet. I tend to look all the time and watch the beauty of the world to feel it. I have learned another way of life, which is feeling life without hearing it.

Discrimination and Accommodations at Work

Discrimination and Reasonable Accommodations Under the Americans with Disabilities Act

Here are few examples that they have on the website, www.nad.org, and it should give you ideas about how you have the right to advocate for yourself and get the accommodations you need.

"Under Title I of the ADA, employers and other covered entities are required to make reasonable accommodation to the physical or mental limitations of an employee:

It is unlawful for a covered entity not to make reasonable accommodation to the known physical or mental limitations of an otherwise qualified applicant or employee with a disability, unless such covered entity can demonstrate that the accommodation would impose an undue hardship on the operation of its business.

.F.R. §1630.9(a). A reasonable accommodation is a modification or adjustment to a job, the work environment, or the way things are usually done to enable a qualified individual with a disability to have an equal employment opportunity. The ADA requires reasonable accommodation: to ensure equal opportunity in the application process, to enable an employee to perform an essential function of a job, and to allow an employee to enjoy equal benefits and privileges of employment.

Reasonable accommodations include telecommunication devices for the deaf (TTYs), video relay service equipment and software, instant messaging software, amplified telephones, visual alarms, assistive listening systems, visible accommodations to communicate audible alarms and messages, and, for deaf employees who rely on sign language, provision of qualified sign language interpreter services. For some individuals and for some jobs, it may be necessary to have interpreter services available on a regular basis. For other employees or for job applicants, occasional interpreting on an as-needed basis may be sufficient. The ADA requires employers to make sure that deaf employees or job applicants can communicate effectively when necessary. This includes special occasions and meetings, training, job evaluations, and communication concerning work, discipline or job benefits. It also includes regular work-related communication and employee-sponsored benefits and programs.

The ADA also requires reasonable transfers of nonessential job duties. For example, a deaf individual would be qualified for a position with a small amount of telephone responsibility, if these responsibilities could be transferred to another employee or handled with a TTY, a TTY relay system, or other accommodation such as e-mail. The regulation specifically lists these accommodations:

Job restructuring; part-time or modified work schedules; reassignment to a vacant position; acquisition or modifications of equipment or devices; appropriate adjustment or modifications of examinations, training materials, or policies; the provision of qualified readers or interpreters; and other similar accommodations for individuals with disabilities.

29 C.F.R. 1630.2(o)(2)(ii). Employers should consult with deaf and hard of hearing employees about the type of accommodations that are needed in order to make its facilities and work environment accessible. The accommodation that is appropriate for one deaf or hard of hearing employee may not be successful in achieving effective communication for other employees.

The duty to provide interpreters and to make other reasonable accommodations is not limited to daily work performance activities or the ability to perform the essential functions of a job. Applicants are entitled to reasonable accommodations during the interview and application process. Employees are entitled to equal access to general information, employee benefits and training opportunities available to other employees. Employees should be able to have access to telephone services, recreational and social activities, emergency procedures, health programs, and the whole range of facilities, services and amenities that are available to other employees. Modifications or adjustments may be required in the work environment, in the manner or circumstances in which a job is customarily performed, and in employment policies."

Every day in America human beings are working around the clock to earn money for their pleasure or to provide income for their families. As you get older, you get used to routine and find a career that you love while making a stepping stone with random jobs that get you to your future. There are thousands of people looking for jobs every day, and they either have numerous years of experience or have graduated from college with a degree. Graduating from high school is a start for income, then a degree from college doubles the income, as education is very important. My mother taught me something that I will always hold in my heart. She says that education is important because if we have war and people come to our country destroying everything we use daily for work and personal use, the only thing they will never destroy is our intelligence, by which she means college education or some kind of certificate that will help you go outside and help to rebuild our community again.

I have gone to college for almost four years; I took a break from education, as I am a mother and have moved a few times. I had a difficult time telling employers that I am deaf and pregnant during my pregnancy, because it is a lot to say and something for them to think about, whether they want to hire me or not. I have if I have a college degree or numerous years of experience with jobs, I would not struggle this much. Even before I was pregnant I applied for jobs before and went to interviews where I struggled and felt discriminated against.

For example, I was in college for three and half years specializing in arts and graphic design, so I created a resume and cover letter that I faxed to the companies. I got phone messages from the answering machine wanting to interview me, as my resume and cover letter was impressive to them. I felt I aced and accomplished the image by making good a presentation already. One woman called and scheduled for me to come in on the following morning; she did not know that I was deaf. So I drove 25 minutes to this place. I was in a business suit and carried a folder with my artwork and paperwork for accommodations the government would provide for me. I walked in, and she was thrilled to see me. She started to walk to get an application form for me to fill out. She was talking while she was walking around her office. I said to her, "Ma'am, I have a hearing loss. I read lips most of the time, but I can still communicate." She shook her head furiously and did not give me the application, as she said it would not work out. I felt hot all of sudden, and battling tears, told myself, *She cannot do this to me, and I am not going to give her an attitude about the way she treated me.* The results did not improve at the end; I ended up staying with her for an hour and half trying to convince her to hire me. She kept asking me questions about my deafness and accommodations. She felt the accommodations would not work for her, and she did not want it in her office. It was frustrating; I left the office and got in my car with tears. I remembered I had another interview in few hours after that, so I kept myself together. I went to my parents, as the second interview was right by their house. My father informed me that the company did not want me to come in, as they found out that I am deaf through calling for me, and my father told them I could not speak on the phone and asked to take a message. They were shocked and told him that it would not work out with my deafness. I bawled and felt like I had failed at the moment.

I even went through a situation few months before where I was working at a company for a month and half. Normally you have to go through training at the training center taking quizzes on the computer and books for at least a week before you go out on the floor. Perhaps I had a difficult time because the computer training. They were animated, like cartoons. I cannot read the lips of cartoon characters, and there was no closed caption provided. John at the time was working there as well, and he was there for a few months before me. He offered to interpret strictly to help me out; some of the people in the human resources had a difficult time accepting that, so I had to do it all alone. On a lighter note, I managed to pass the tests after taking it over and over again. After a week of training and several hours of taking the tests, I was put out on the floor. Again, the normal way is that employees wear their apron and a button that says that they are in training for a week at the most. My department decided that I should not wear an apron yet, so I wore the button. However I spent a month on the floor with the button and never got to wear the apron. I went through many humiliating experiences on the floor where people that I worked with disrespected me. I had years of experiences with walking around forklifts, as my father owned a flooring business for 30 years and had forklifts, carpets, and other stuff around the warehouse. I assisted the people using the forklift when I walked 15 feet ahead of it to make sure the aisles were clear a few times without a hassle. However, one day my department manager came up running to me screaming at the top of her lungs, "You cannot do this! You cannot hear. No, no, no, stop!" She continued to yell at me in front of customers and other employees. She even yelled at the guy who was using the forklift. He told her I had assisted him a couple of times and did fine, so he trusted me with it. I felt hurt and disrespected by her. They put me in the desk area and had me stock things on the floor, any time that customer came up to me for assistance, an employee rushed to tell them that I could not help them for personal reasons.

One afternoon I was finally doing work where I was helping this woman with interior design by ordering window blinds and entering the order in the computer. I spent an hour with her; I clarified on a lot of things to make sure we were on the same level so I would not mess up on the order. She was telling me that she was impressed with me and my skills, so I finally felt I was on the right path. The next thing I knew, an older man who had been there for years pushed my chair that had wheels on it, wheeling me away, and informed the customer that I could not do it because of my deafness. The woman kept telling him that I was doing great, and we were finishing up the order. He finished the order with over five grand and put it in his name instead of mine. He went outside to smoke. As John overheard him talking about what he did John was furious and found me at work as I was about to clock out. But I had to finish up cleaning the area. The guy asked me if I wanted to finish his order, which was 10 bucks worth of Disney wall paper. He laughed.

On my way out to clock out, I asked my department manager when would I be able to wear the apron, as I had been there for almost two months. She said it would be awhile. John saw everything that was going on to me on that day and decided it was time to walk out. I regret not reporting the companies, like the two specific companies to prevent discrimination in the future. I felt I had a lack of evidence, and my family felt I should not fight it, as it would be greedy to get money from the government, so I left it alone. So if any of you go through discrimination, please have the courage to report it, and you will be helping out by preventing them from discriminating future people. Also, it would be wise to get education and complete it to show them your skills instead them looking at you and judging you immediately.

Also, work with good companies who respect you for who you are where they are willing to communicate with you and meet your needs. I have had a few jobs that respected me, and we had a system of communication. For example, I informed the staff not to talk to me in the kennel where we are feeding dogs and cleaning their kennels. It gets very loud, as the dogs beg to get out to play in the yard and away from other dogs' barking. When you get to the hallway outside of the kennel it gets quieter. I told them that they could talk to me out in the hallway first before we teamed up to help each other to go in the kennels. My boss had meetings every month; we would talk about communication, and I would come up with the suggestions so we could work as a team on good terms. I even told my boss to write out the guidelines of what she was going to talk about, so I knew ahead of time what she was talking about when it came to work and staff.

I also worked at a retail clothing store. I had very nice bosses. They helped me with customers when I told them I could not go to fitting rooms and knock on their doors to ask if they need anything because I could not hear them. They were fine and did it for me sometimes or let me be a cashier. We all worked out a system. Also, I worked for rafting company in California for a summer. There were two store locations. The office would call one of the store locations to notify us when the customers were coming or to book more trips, etc. Kate and I were lucky, because we had the photographers, rafting guides, or other bus drivers that would kindly answer the phones for us.

Overall, do not let discrimination or lack of help stop you to get what you need for work performance. There are people out there who discriminate against not only deaf people; they discriminate based on sexual orientation, race, appearance, health problems, like HIV or learning disabilities. Some employers and schools disrespect their staff and students. I was told by my family that they are just busy picking on others as they have low self esteem and do not like themselves. They want to have power to control others with their attitude of discrimination. I find it strange that people talk to others that are different from the norm in areas such as race, sexual orientation, or in a disrespectful manner.

The Dalai Lama once said, "From the viewpoint of absolute truth, what we feel and experience in our ordinary daily life is all delusion. Of all the various delusions, the sense of discrimination between oneself and others is the worst form, as it creates nothing but unpleasantness." My father said to me that if I quit, I would never see my strengths after achieving something. He told me I need to be strong, because this world is huge, and I have to battle the challenges. He told me not to give up on things even if it takes several times to get up to perfect the way I want it to be. Bill Clinton said "If you live long enough, you will make mistakes. But if you learn from them, you will be a better person. It is how you handle adversity, not how it affects you. The main thing is never quit, never quit, never quit."

My childhood best friend was a screenwriter for a television show; my other best friend was a rafting guide for class-two to class-four rapids, where she was responsible for lives in her boat out on the rapids. Also, she is certified forklift driver. Her close friends are teachers at the deaf school. There are doctors out there; they have nurses that wear clear mask so they can lip read them during surgery. "High achievers spot rich opportunities swiftly, make big decisions quickly and move into action immediately. Follow these principles and you can make your dreams come true," said Robert H. Schuller.

Do not let anyone stop your dreams, passion, and you becoming whom you are. You have the right to aim at what you want to do with your life. There will be people out there who will doubt you; you will have to work hard, as the character, Andy did in the movie, *The Devil Wears Prada,* proving to her boss, Miranda, that she was a capable, hard worker, and Miranda would not regret having her in her office. If you tend to work hard to prove others what you are cable of, you will feel excellent about yourself. Here are several quotes.

"Shoot for the moon. Even if you miss, you'll land among the stars."
~Les Brown

"Go confidently in the direction of your dreams. Live the life you have imagined." ~Henry David Thoreau

"Courage is resistance to fear, mastery of fear—not absence of fear." ~Mark Twain

"Courage is the most important of all the virtues, because without courage you can't practice any other virtue consistently. You can practice any virtue erratically, but nothing consistently without courage." ~Maya Angelou

Accepting Myself

As I stand here on the gravity of this Earth, I watch the beauty of life where I see the nature of what the world has created for us to see and listen to. I listen with my soul to feel the beauty of life with or without sounds. I enter a page every morning of my life where God has written a book for me to test the waters and overcome the challenges he puts in my life to test my strengths and weakness. I am forever grateful for all the lessons he has taught me as I have accepted who I am. He did a life map for me to learn to listen my soul and do something positive daily, as I appreciate what he has provided me, such as my family, my daughter, John, my best friends, and the rest. Everything happens for a reason. Where I do not know why he gives me a challenge when I face it, then after I achieve and master the challenge, I soon will realize why he wanted me to experience a situation along the deaf journey he gifted me with. To succeed in life is to accept yourself. You have to love who you are and the life you have at the moment. Even when things get bad, there will be a light at the end of the tunnel for you to reach after you battle the hard times. When that occurs, you get stronger and feel confident that you have healed the moments, and you find the happiness again.

Accepting myself gives me great deal of confidence. I can trust the world in God's hands because I would not be where I am at if I did not experience this deaf journey of mine. I am truly blessed to have this opportunity that he has given me. I am a sensitive young lady who learned how to feel life without sounds and connect with it. Of course, I enjoy having the power in controlling what sounds I want to hear and what I do not want to hear! I enjoy that I have an ability to hear music, the animals making noises in our environment, my daughter cooing and laughing in her sleep, and hear the water running down the river as I stand and be calm. My deafness has reached the point where I care for others and long to help them. I love to be there for my family and friends whenever they need to vent and have someone to listen as I really have to, since I lip read them! Obviously, I am an excellent listener. I tend to be sensitive, as I am a care giver for my grandmother while being a mother to my daughter. I even had a haircut, and I had my hairdresser cut 13 inches off of my hair to give it to my best friend's cousin who was diagnosed with cancer. I absolutely love her family, as I love and care for my best friend who has been there for me through thick and thin. She is Godmother of my daughter.

I listen to the world and trust life by accepting who I am. I do not do well in the darkness where I often have to say, "Turn the lights on; I can't hear you," if I have to respond to my loved ones. I never want them to think I do not care, and I don't want to look like a fool if I do not understand, so I communicate with the lights on. Think about how you connect with your pet who cannot even speak. You feel it as you touch and watch how it interacts with you while it shows some kind of personality and how it feels. This is how I am attentive to the world when I go grocery shopping and watch people shop for their families or when someone is voicing an opinion. Another perfect example is music videos; they have actors and actresses being silent and express the song as a story while you listen to the singer. You understand the story line by watching them expressing their feelings without their voice their emotions. I have adapted to the silent world and manage to survive in the hearing world.

Also, I had to work harder than other kids my own age to survive and keep up with life. I did not really have a playful childhood; I did a lot of sports, as I was lucky enough to find the time away from doing speech therapy and tutoring. I am happy that I am a mother. I can relive my childhood again by watching cartoons with closed captions, as back in my younger days I was not able to watch cartoons because

I could not understand the characters. I am able to read stories to her as my mother read several stories to me; I focused on the pictures then, as I was not able to understand what she read to me. I am able to play games that I did not get to learn. I am able to learn the traditional songs as we would have to teach her. With the speech therapy and tutoring, it has shaped me into who I am today, as I worked hard. My parents would tell me often that they wonder if they should have just let me learn sign language, because I am a chatterbox. When I share my updates with them I like to share every detail of it. They would have a difficult time to go to sleep, as I would continue to ramble about the events. Then they would turn the lights off, hoping I would end the conversation. Of course I would turn the lights on and tell them, "I cannot hear your response in the dark. This trick will not get me to end my conversations!'

Another great thing is that my life is rather entertaining; it is filled with love and laughter. I make a lot of jokes, because I really cannot understand jokes, so I make up my own jokes, like, "How do you say spaghetti in Spanish? Spaghettios!" When I was a little girl my mother said to me that when she had a run in her stockings, I asked her, "Mom, stockings can run?" as I take words literally. Even When people ask me if I understood what someone said, like the radio or speaker, I kid myself and say, "And you are asking me? You are asking a deaf person?" then they realize it was silly of them to ask me that. I continue to learn how to pronounce correctly. I prefer to learn a word pronounced the way it actually was spelled. I absolutely find it tricky to pronounce words that are not pronounced the way they are spelled, for example, "Hola." I could have pronounced it as "holla" or "ho-la" instead of "ola."

I could have bad days and come home, and they would ask me how was my day. I would say, "I had to start my day over several times today." I believe if I am having a bad day because I have a problem with my deafness or a situation related to my deafness, I will start my day again after an hour goes by, when it is a new hour for me to begin.

I have to picture sunlight in my mind as a way to maintain a positive attitude bout my life, to keep on being strong and holding the ropes to climb up the mountain. I shall not sweat small or big stuff while I learn how to handle things with grace and a good attitude, because it is not worth the stress to dwell on the stuff. I try to live as if it is the last day of my life, meaning, I try to make the best outcome of my day. What doesn't kill you makes you stronger; I have had days where I felt my heart was broken into pieces, and I would gather the pieces back together as a puzzle.

I am content with the direction of my life. I am at ease with the results I have seen, and I am happy to know who I am and being confident as a young deaf woman. I enjoy writing poems to express thoughts through my deafness. As I stand still and see the world moving with emotions, my thoughts continuously travel through the poetry of art and emotions. Obviously, I am a sensitive young woman who has been through a lot and learned how to overcome my challenges. I become my own advocate when I walk out of my home to get in the car and face the hearing world. I do not give up on life, and I forgive others, because life is short, and I am the type of person who does not want to look back and ponder what ifs. I trust the road where my journey is going to take me in the future because I have accepted life and most of all, myself.

I love being deaf and cannot wait to learn more about myself as I get older and enter several new chapters of my life. I have faith and confidence, which is what gets me by in life. What is amazing is that I wished on a star every night during the summers in Vermont, wondering about my life. My heart was full of passion and hopeful for the future. Now I look at my life today; I have experienced tremendously wonderful things, even though there were many tears in my life. I am blessed for the bad times, even though that sounds strange, but it made me stronger. I never thought I would be playing sports, but it turned out I was good at basketball and cheerleading. I never thought I would have great friends, but have great friends. I have a wonderful family who raised me and supported me greatly. Last, I am a deaf mother of my daughter. I am addicted to her angelic movements when she is sleepy or when she giggles at small things in life. I got to this road because I never gave up trying to figure out who I am and accepting my life, which is being deaf. I look forward to what the future has to offer me.

The Road to Life
By Ashlee Holland

From the sunrise, it's a new beautiful day.
Going out into a world full of challenges that we must conquer daily
Whether they are small or big
Whether we succeed or fail
Failing at our obstacles is out of the question;
We must continue to strive for our dreams.
As the wind blows, we shall follow wherever the wind takes us
Putting faith in our hands and letting it take us to life,
Just like a butterfly travels around, fluttering in spirit,
All it takes is strength in our blood to battle the challenges.
Your soul is full of gold and happiness
Each day you shall be grateful for what life offers
As a door opens to another,
Your journey guides you where you are supposed to be.
Life is meant to be a path for you to find out who you are.
Enjoy the spills and thrills of life, as life is short.
Accepting yourself is the greatest key to success
Confidence is a key to turn a new chapter in life.
Don't give up!
Be kind to others, learn something from others,
Always remember to try to forgive.

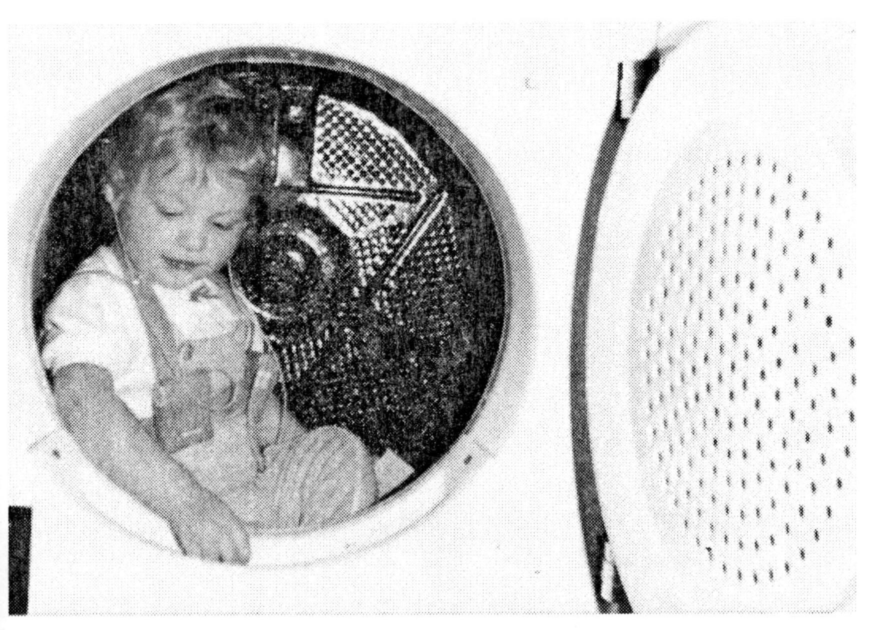

Ashlee with her hearing aids. Age 2.

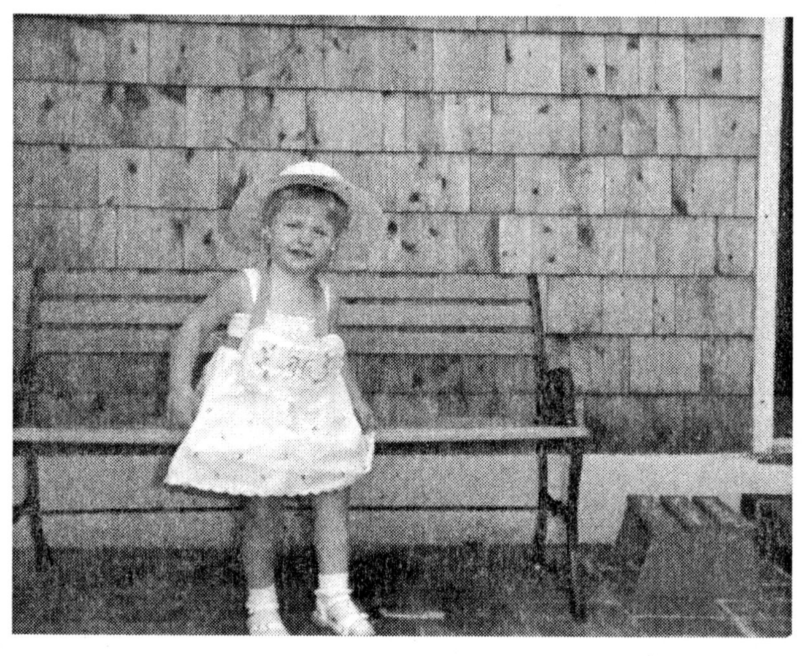

Ashlee wearing fashion pouch for her hearing aids. Age 2.

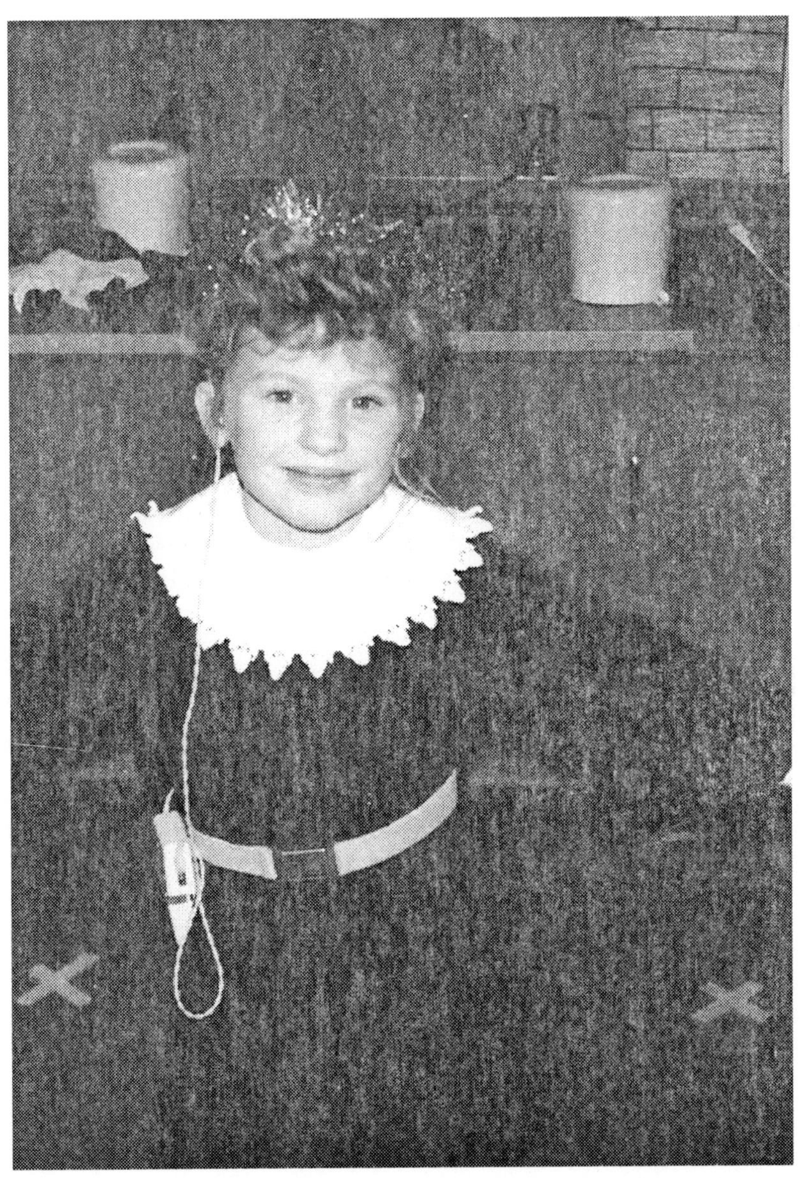

Ashlee wearing her FM system in class. Age 4.

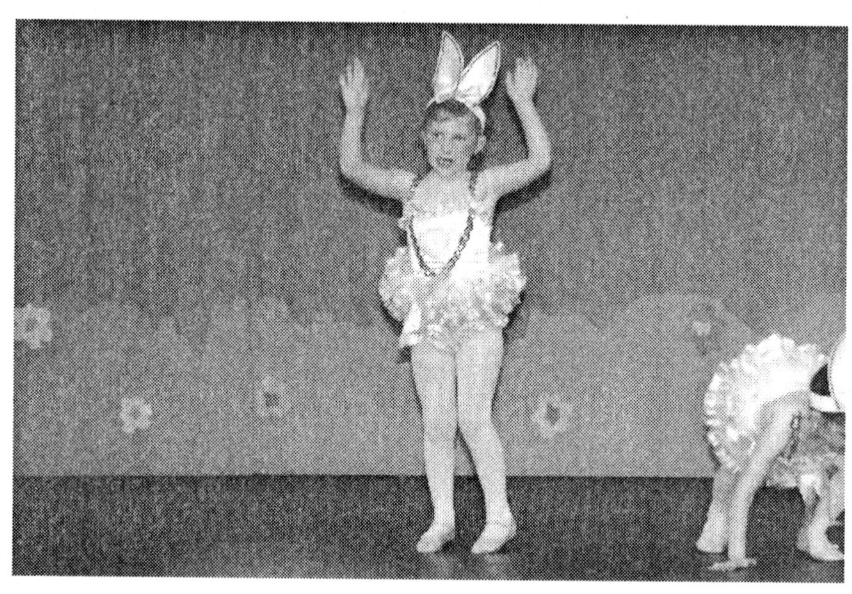

Dance recital in Vermont. Age 4.

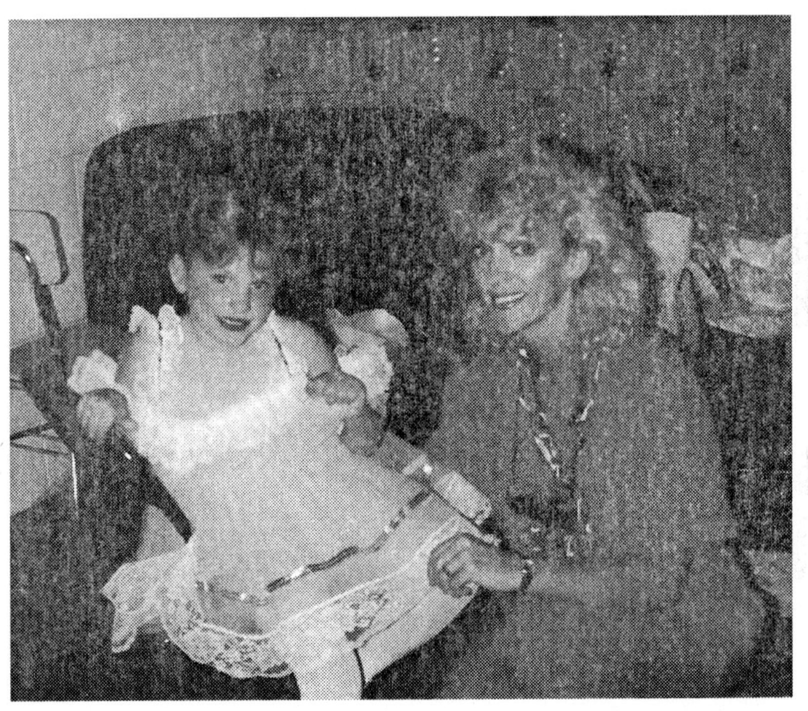

Ashlee and her mother at a dance recital. Age 4.

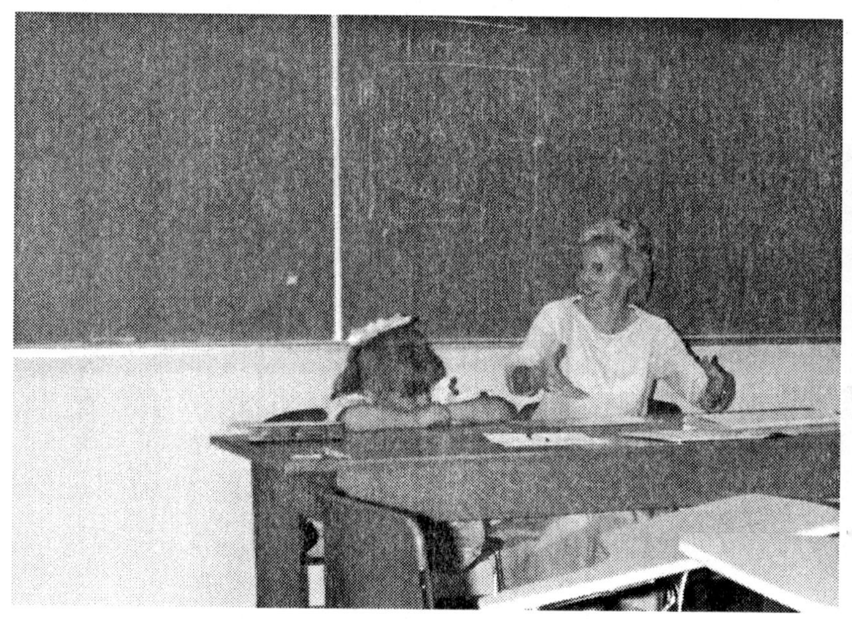

Sandy "Ba Ba" and Ashlee. Age 4.

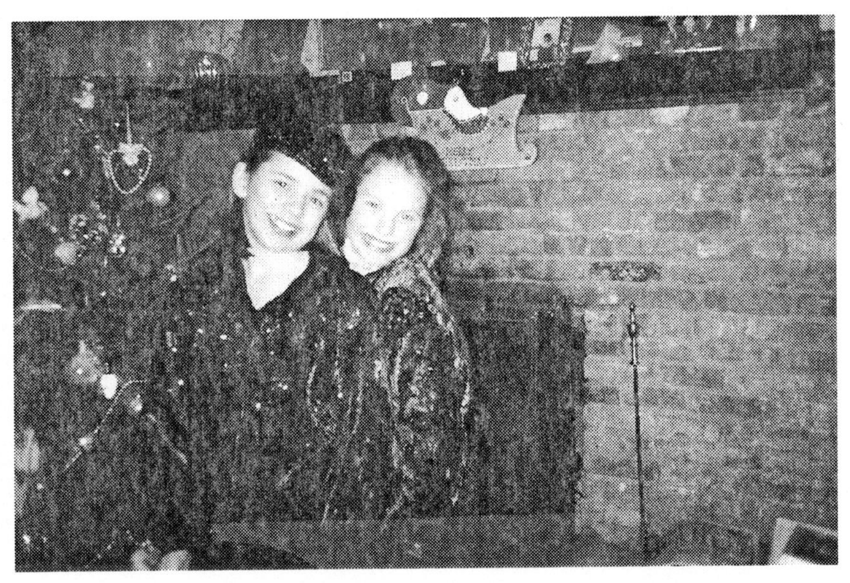

Ashlee and her deaf friend Ally in Beverly, Ma. Age 8.

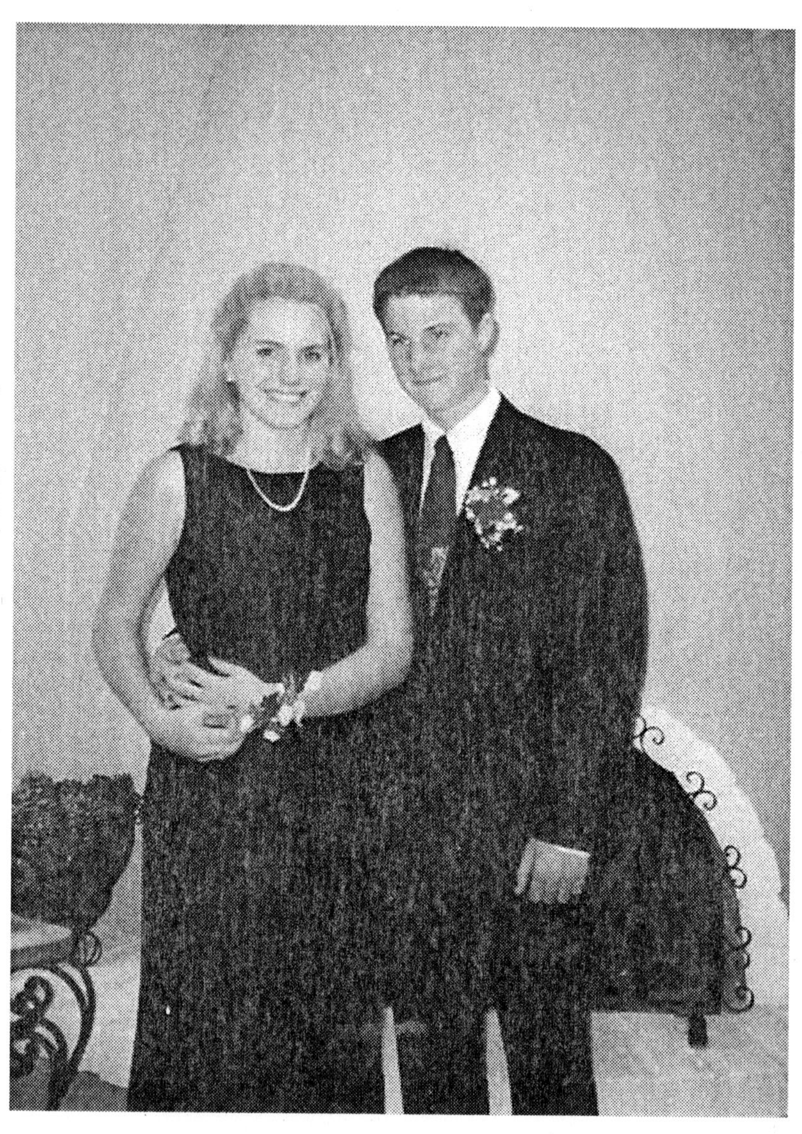

Ashlee's first high school dance. Age 15.

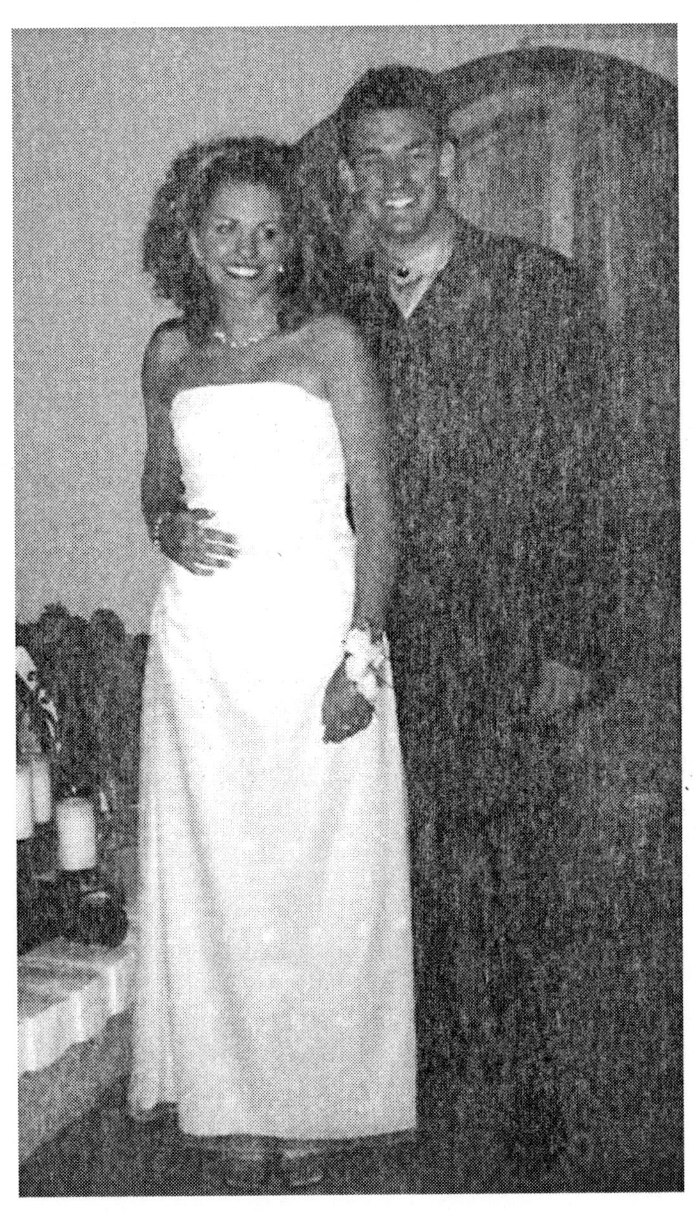

Ashlee's first prom. Age 17.

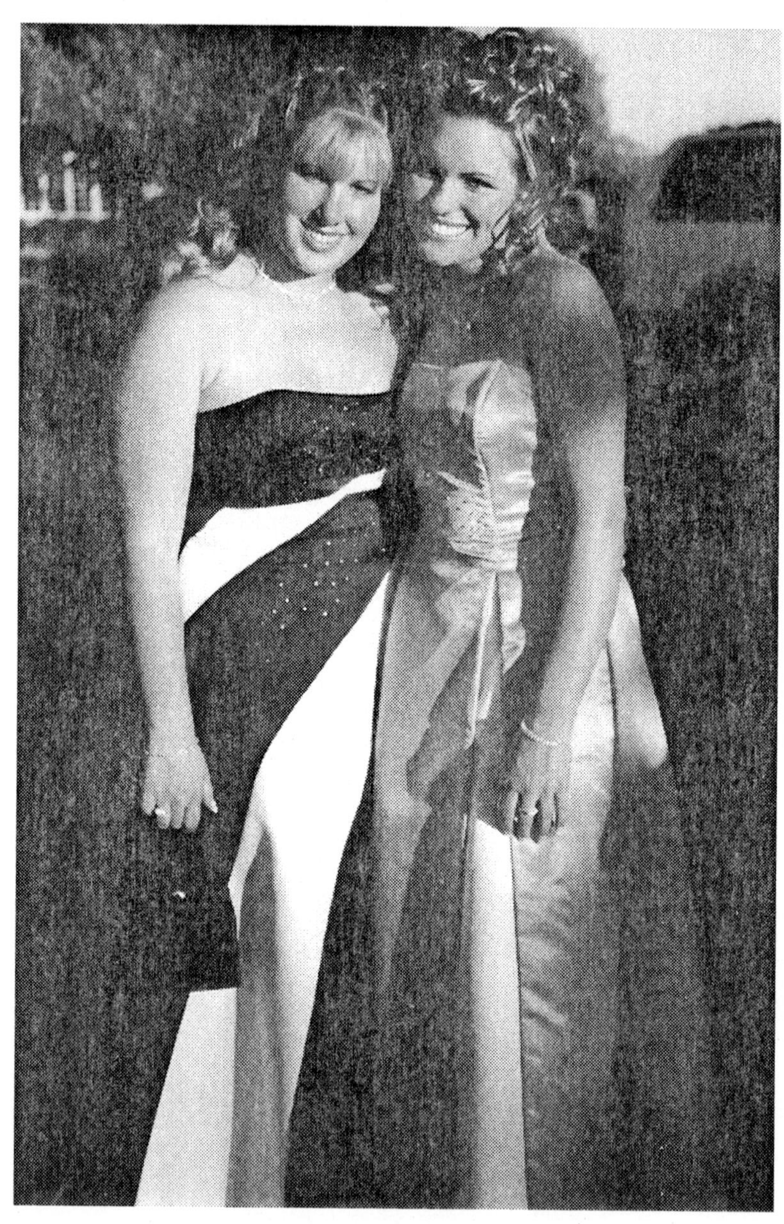

Ashlee and Brooke at their senior prom .

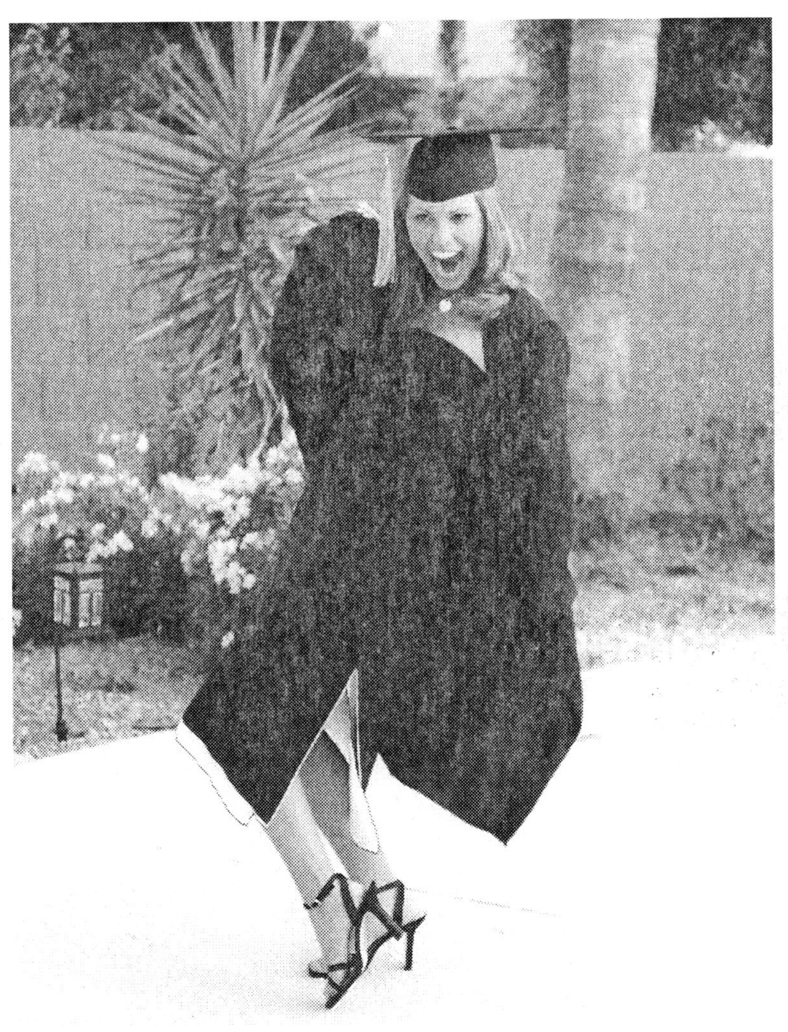

High school graduation. Age 18.

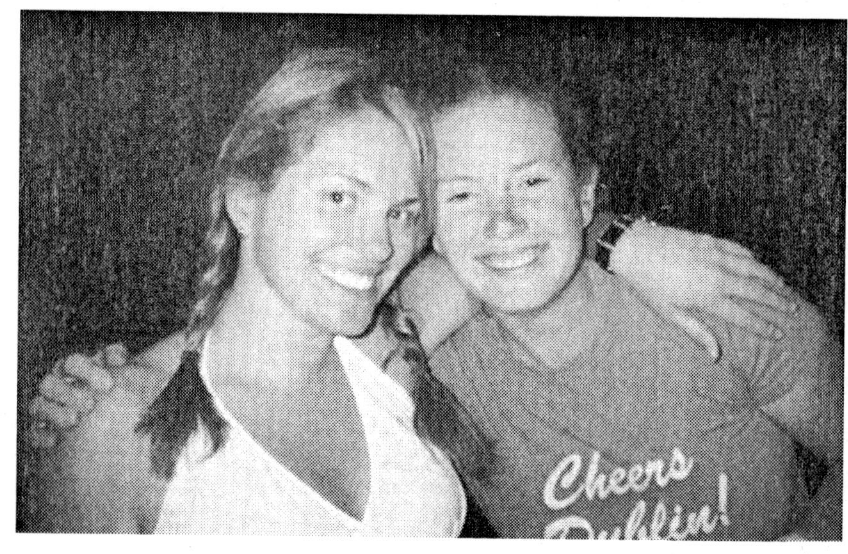

Ashlee and her deaf friend, Kate who introduced me
to ASL. Age 20.

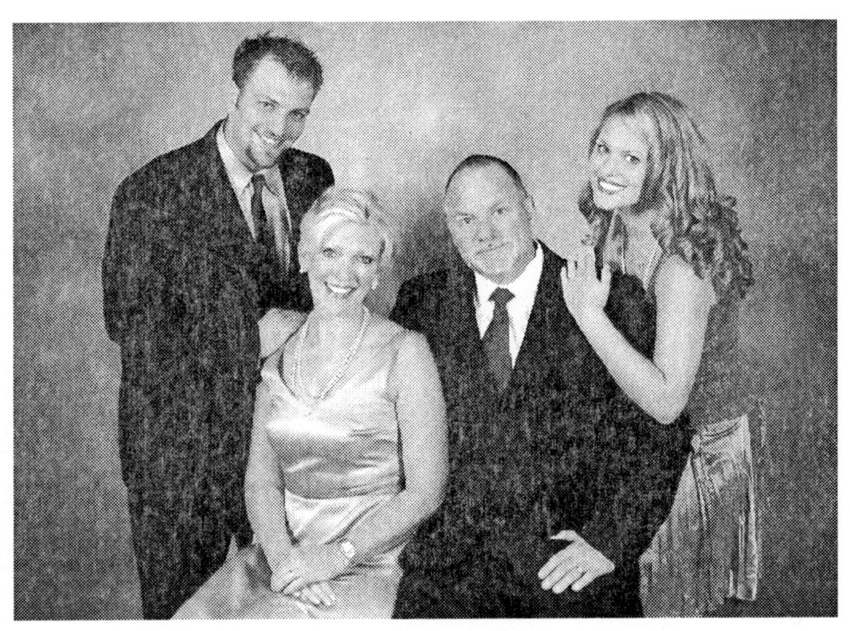

Ashlee's family portrait in Alaska. Age 21.

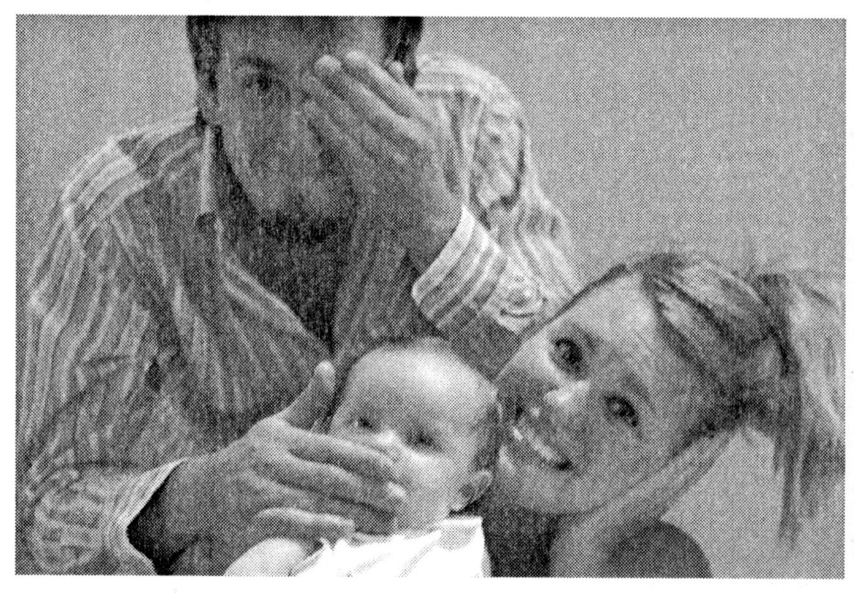

Hear No Evil, See No Evil, Speak No Evil.

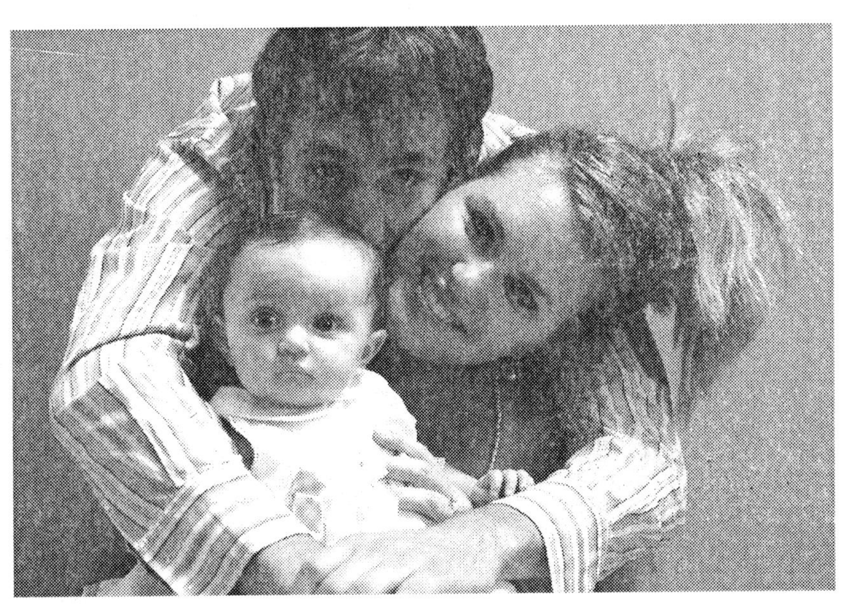

John, Makayla Rose, and Ashlee. Age 23.